MW00445514

SOCIAL INTEREST:

A CHALLENGE TO MANKIND

by

ALFRED ADLER

translated by
John Linton, M.A., *and*
Richard Vaughan

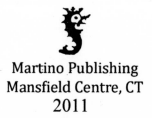

Martino Publishing
Mansfield Centre, CT
2011

Martino Publishing
P.O. Box 373,
Mansfield Centre, CT 06250 USA

www.martinopublishing.com

ISBN   978-1-61427-082-9

© 2011 Martino Publishing

All rights reserved. No new contribution to this publication may
be reproduced, stored in a retrieval system, or transmitted, in any form or
by any means, electronic, mechanical, photocopying, recording, or otherwise,
without the prior permission of the Publisher.

Cover design by T. Matarazzo

Printed in the United States of America On 100% Acid-Free Paper

SOCIAL INTEREST:

A CHALLENGE TO MANKIND

by

ALFRED ADLER

translated by
John Linton, M.A., *and*
Richard Vaughan

FABER AND FABER LTD
24 Russell Square
London

FIRST PUBLISHED IN MAY MCMXXXVIII
BY FABER AND FABER LIMITED

'Man knows much more than he understands.'
—ADLER

CONTENTS

9

PREFACE

In the course of my life as consultant physician in cases of mental illnesses and in clinics, as a psychologist and teacher in schools and in families, I have had constant opportunity of surveying a vast amount of human material. I made it strictly my business never to make any statement I could not illustrate and prove from my own experience. It is not surprising that in doing this I came occasionally into conflict with the preconceived ideas of other men who in many cases could only study our human lot much less intensively. When this happened I endeavoured to examine dispassionately the essential arguments of other investigators. I could do this the more easily since I believe I am not bound by any strict rule or prepossession, but rather subscribe to the maxim: Everything can be something else as well. The uniqueness of the individual cannot be expressed in a short formula, and general rules—even those laid down by Individual Psychology, which I have created —should be nothing more than an aid to a preliminary illumination of a field of vision on which the single individual can be found—or missed. The value thus assigned to rules—the stronger emphasis laid on flexibility and on empathy with shades of difference—has every time strengthened my conviction with regard to the free creative power of the individual in his earliest childhood, and his restricted power in later life, when the child has already adopted a fixed law of movement for his life. According to this view, which allows the child free scope for his struggle for perfection, fulfilment, mastery, or evolution, one can look upon the influences of environment and upbringing as the materials with which the child in play constructs his style of life.

And still another conviction was forced upon me. The construction of the child's style of life has to be rightly carried out *sub specie aeternitatis*, if it is to stand the tests life imposes without suffering any set-backs. The child is constantly confronted afresh with ever-varying problems that cannot be solved either by trained (conditioned) reflexes or by innate psychical capacities. It would be a most hazardous venture to expose a child equipped only with trained reflexes or with innate capacities to the tests of a world that is continually raising new problems. There would always be waiting in reserve the most difficult problem to be solved by the unresting, creative spirit which is definitely impelled to follow the path of the child's style of life. Everything that has a name in the various schools of psychology takes the same course—instincts, impulses, feeling, thinking, action, the attitude to pleasure and pain, and finally self-love and social feeling. The style of life takes command of all expressive forms—the whole rules the parts. If an error is present it is found in the law of movement, in the final goal of the style of life and not in any partial expression of it.

A third fact this investigation has impressed upon me: every semblance of causality in the psychical life is due to the tendency of many psychologists to present their dogmas disguised in mechanistic or physical similes. At one time they use as a comparison a pump-handle moving up and down, at another a magnet with polar termini, at another a sadly harassed animal struggling for the satisfaction of its elementary needs. It is plain that from a standpoint like this few of the fundamental varieties shown by man's psychical life can be observed. Since physical science has taken the ground of causality from under the feet of psychologists and in place of it speaks in favour of a statistical probability in the issue of events, then surely the attacks on Individual Psychology for its denial of causality in psychical events need no longer be taken seriously. It may possibly be clear even to the layman that the millionfold variations of faulty actions can be 'understood' as faulty actions, but cannot be comprehended causally.

When we now rightly leave the ground of absolute certitude, on which so many psychologists bustle about, there remains for us only one single standard by which we can form an estimate of a human being—*his movement when confronted with the unavoidable problems of humanity.* Three problems are irrevocably set before every individual. These are—the attitude taken up towards our

THE MEASURE OF HUMANS

THE INDIVIDUAL IS PART OF THE WHOLE

WHAT IS ONE'S ATTITUDE TOWARD OTHERS?
TOWARD VOCATION?
TOWARD LOVE?

PREFACE

fellow men, vocation, and love. All three are linked with one another by the first; they are not casual questions; they are inevitable. They arise from the relationship of man to human society, to the cosmic factors, and to the other sex. Their solution decides the destiny and the welfare of humanity. Man is a part of the whole. His value, too, depends on his individual solution of these problems. They can be regarded as a mathematical task that has to be undertaken. The worse the failure, the more numerous are the complications that threaten the possessor of a faulty style of life. These complications seem to be absent only so long as the reliability of his social feeling is not put to the proof. The exogenous factor—the nearness of the task that demands co-operation and fellowship—is always the cause of the symptoms that give evidence of the mistake; these are difficulty of upbringing, neurosis and psycho-neurosis, suicide, crime, addiction to drugs, and sexual perversions.

If the maladjustment to social life is thus unmasked, then the question arises—and this is not merely an academic question but one of vital importance for the cure —how and when has the growth of social feeling been drained of its strength? In our search for events that will provide an adequate explanation we happen on the period of earliest childhood and on situations which, as experience shows, are able to effect a hindrance to the proper development. But the discovery of this hindrance is always accompanied by the child's faulty response to it. And on a closer examination of the circumstances that come to light it is seen that at one time a legitimate

14

The core challenge of education — to teach co-operation and interest in other persons

interference has received a faulty response, at another time a mistaken interference has received a wrong response, and at a third time—though this is far less frequent—a mistaken interference has received a correct response. It is also seen that further steps were taken in this direction, which always has conquest for its goal, without the opposing influences having led to the abandonment of the path that has once been chosen. Accordingly education, however widely one may fix its boundaries, means not only allowing favourable influences to have their effect, but also ascertaining exactly what the creative power of the child has formed out of them, in order afterwards to smooth the path to improvement in the case of faulty formation. This better way is found in every case to be the increase of co-operation and of interest in other persons.

Once the child has found his law of movement, in which there must be noted the rhythm, the temperament, the activity, and above all the degree of social feeling—phenomena that can often be recognized even in the second year and without fail in the fifth—then all his other capacities with their particular trends are also linked with these to this law of movement. This work will deal chiefly with the apperception connected with this law of movement—the way in which man looks at himself and the external world. In other words we shall deal with the conception which the child, and later, on the same lines, the adult, has acquired of himself and the world. Further, this meaning cannot be gathered from the words and thoughts of the person

15

under examination. These are all far too strongly under the spell of the law of movement, which aims at conquest, and therefore even in the case of self-condemnation still casts longing glances towards the heights. Of greater importance is the fact that life in its wholeness, named concretely by me, 'style of life', is built up by the child at a time when he has neither language nor ideas adequate to give it expression. If he develops further in his intelligence he does so in a movement that has never been comprehended in words and is therefore not open to the assaults of criticism; it is even withdrawn from the criticism of experience. There can be no question here of anything like a repressed unconscious; it is rather a question of something not understood, of something withheld from the understanding. But man speaks to the adept with his style of living and with his reaction to the problems of life, which demand social feeling for their solution.

So far then as man's meaning about himself and about the external world is concerned, this can be best discovered from the significance he finds in life and from the significance he gives to his own life. It is obvious that here possible discord with an ideal social feeling, with social life, co-operation, and the sense of fellowship can be distinctly heard.

We are now prepared to understand how important it is to get to know something of the meaning of life and also to discover the conceptions different people have of this meaning. If there exists, at least to some extent, a reliable knowledge of that meaning of life which lies beyond the scope of our own experience, then it is clear that this puts those persons in the wrong who flagrantly contradict it.

As will be seen, the author is modest enough to endeavour to obtain at the start a partial success which seems to him to be borne out by his experiences. He undertakes this task all the more willingly since he cherishes the hope that with a somewhat fuller knowledge of the meaning of life, not only will a scientific programme be matured for further investigation along the lines he has laid down, but also that with growing knowledge there will be a notable increase in the number of those who can be won over to accept this meaning of life by a better understanding of it.

CHAPTER I

THE CONCEPTION OF ONESELF
AND THE WORLD

For me there can be no doubt that every individual conducts himself in life as if he had a definite idea of his power and his capacities, and also as though from the very beginning he had a clear conception of the difficulty or feasibility of his action in any given case. In a word, I am convinced that *a person's behaviour springs from his idea*. We should not be surprised at this, because our senses do not receive actual facts, but merely a subjective image of them—a reflection of the external world. *Omnia ad opinionem suspensa sunt.* This saying of Seneca's should not be forgotten in psychological investigations. How we interpret the great and important facts of existence depends upon our style of life. Only at the point where we come directly up against facts that reveal a contradiction to our interpretation are we inclined in our immediate experience to correct our view of them in minor details, and allow the law of causality to influence us without changing our conception of life. As a matter of fact, it has the same effect on me whether a poisonous snake is actually approaching my foot or whether I merely believe that it is a poisonous snake. The spoiled child shows entirely the same anxiety whether he is afraid of burglars as soon as his mother leaves him or whether there are really burglars in the house. In either case he keeps to his opinion that he cannot exist without his mother, even when the supposition that has roused his anxiety has been proved to be wrong. The man who suffers from agoraphobia and avoids the street because he feels and believes that the ground is swaying beneath his feet, could not behave in any other way if, during his periods of health, the ground beneath his feet were actually swaying. The burglar who shuns useful work because he mistakenly finds burgling easier owing to his being unprepared for co-operation, can show the same disinclination for work when it would really be harder than housebreaking. A suicide finds death preferable to a life which he assumes is hopeless. He could act in the same way if his life were really hopeless. The drug-addict obtains from his poison a relief which he values more highly than the honourable solution of his life's problems. He could act in the same way if this were really valid for him. The homosexual man is afraid of women and finds them unattractive, while men, whose conquest seems to him to be a triumph, allure him. All these act at times according to a belief which, if it were correct, would make their behaviour objectively right.

Take the following case: a barrister of thirty-six has lost all interest in his work. He is unsuccessful and attributes this to the fact that he does not make a good impression on the few clients who come to consult him. He always found great difficulty as well in mixing with other people, and, especially in the company of girls, he was always extremely shy. A marriage, into which he entered with great reluctance, indeed with aversion, ended a year later in a divorce. He now lives quite withdrawn from the world in the house of his parents, who have for the most part to provide for him.

He is an only child and he was spoiled by his mother to an incredible extent. She was always with him. She succeeded in convincing both the child and his father that he would one day become a very outstanding man. The boy grew up with this expectation, and his brilliant success at school seemed to confirm it. As commonly happens with most spoiled children, who can deny themselves nothing, childish masturbation gained a harmful mastery over him and soon made him the laughing-stock of the girls in the school, who had discovered his secret misdemeanour. He withdrew from them entirely. In his isolation he abandoned himself to the imagination of achieving the most glorious triumphs in love and marriage; but he felt himself attracted only to his mother, whom he completely dominated, and with whom for a considerable time he connected his sexual fantasies. It is also obvious enough from this case that this so-called Oedipus complex is not a 'fundamental fact', but is simply a vicious unnatural result of maternal over-indulgence. This comes more clearly into view when the boy or the youth in his inordinate vanity sees himself betrayed by girls and has not developed sufficient social interest to be able to mix with other people.

Shortly before finishing his studies, when faced with the question of gaining an independent livelihood, the patient was seized with melancholia, so that now once again he beat a retreat. Like all pampered children he was timid as a child and drew back from strangers. Later the same thing happened with his comradeships in the case both of men and women. In the same way he drew back from his career, and this situation, only slightly modified, persists up to the present.

I content myself with this statement, omitting the other facts that are in accordance with it—the 'reasons', the excuses, and the other pathological symptoms with which he 'secured' his retreat. One thing is clear: this man never altered throughout his whole life. He always wanted to be first and invariably drew back whenever he was uncertain of success. His idea of life—hidden from him, but conjectured by us—can be expressed in this form: 'Since the world withholds my triumph from me, I will retreat.' It cannot be denied that as a man who sees in his triumph over others the completion for which he has striven, he has in this way acted only rightly and intelligently. There is no 'reason', no 'common sense' in the law of movement he has given himself, but rather what I have termed 'private intelligence'. If as a matter of fact it were denied that this kind of life could be of *any* value to any one, he would act in very much the same way.

The following case seems similar to this, only it has different expressive forms and is less hampered by the tendency to switch off from other people. A man of twenty-six grew up as the second child between two other members of his family, whom his mother preferred to him. With great jealousy he set himself to rival the superior performances of his elder brother. He adopted a critical attitude towards his mother and depended on his father—always a second phase in the life of a child. His aversion to his mother extended before long to the entire female sex as a result of the intolerable habits of his grandmother and a nurse. His ambition to be rid of the rule of women and to dominate men increased enormously. He tried in every way to undermine his brother's superior position. The brother's advantage over him in bodily strength, in gymnastics, and in hunting made him hate all forms of physical exercise. He excluded these from the sphere of his activity, just as he was already on the point of eliminating women. Achievements attracted him only if they were linked for him with a sense of triumph. For a considerable time he was in love with a girl and adored her from a very great distance. Evidently this aloofness did not please the girl and she discarded him in favour of another man. His brother had made a happy marriage and this made him afraid that he would be less fortunate, and that he would again play a secondary part in the opinion of the world, as he had done before in childhood with his mother. I will give one example among many of his urge to dispute this brother's superiority. On one occasion the brother returned from hunting with a fine fox pelt, of which he was very proud. Our friend secretly cut off the white brush in order to nullify his brothers' triumph. His sexual instinct, in view of its greater activity within narrower limits, took the only direction that remained after his elimination of women and it became homosexual. His interpretation of the meaning of life was easy to decipher. Life means: I must be the superior in everything I undertake. And he endeavoured to attain this superiority by excluding all actions in which he felt he could not achieve a triumphal fulfilment. The first bitter and troubling fact he had to acknowledge in the course of our conversations that were meant to throw light on his case was the claim his partner in homosexual intercourse also made to a victory which was due to his magical power of attraction.

With regard to this case as well we may assert that the 'private intelligence' was not at fault and that most people would follow the same course if refusal on the part of girls were a universal truth. In fact a strong tendency to generalize occurs very frequently as a fundamental error in the construction of a style of life.

'Life-plan' and 'meaning'[1] mutually supplement one another. Both have their roots in a period when the child is incapable of drawing inferences from his experience and expressing them in words and concepts. He has, however, already begun to develop more general forms for his behaviour from inferences that are not expressed in words, from events that are often insignificant, or from experiences not expressed in words that

[1] *Lebensplan* and *Meinung*; *Meinung* here means 'the idea one has of life'.

24

are strongly charged with emotion. These general inferences, with their corresponding tendencies, formed at a
time when words and concepts are lacking, continue to
have their effect in later years, although they are certainly modified in various ways; common sense intervenes to correct them to a greater or less extent and is
able to keep people from relying too much on rules,
phrases, and principles. As we shall see later, we owe
to common sense, enhanced by social feeling, this libera-
tion from the excessive effort to find support and security
which results from an oppressive sense of insecurity and
inferiority.

The following case, which is one that may be frequently observed, shows that the same mistaken process
is found in animals as well. A puppy was being trained
to follow his master in the street. After making fairly
good progress in this art it occurred to him one day to
jump into a moving car. He was flung off from the car
without being injured. This was certainly a unique
experience, for which he could scarcely have an innate
reaction ready. It would be difficult also to speak of a
'conditioned reflex' when one learns that this dog, while
making further progress in his training, could no longer
be induced to approach the place of the accident. He
was afraid neither of streets nor of vehicles but of the
place of the accident, and made the same general infer-
ence as human beings often make—that the place and
not his own carelessness and inexperience was to blame.
And danger *always* threatened him on this spot. He was
like many others who adopt a similar procedure. They

cling fast to such interpretations because in doing so they make sure at least of one thing—they can never again be injured 'on this spot'. Similar structures occur frequently in neurosis. The neurotic person fears a threatened defeat—a loss of his sense of individuality—and tries to protect himself by making the best of the physical or psychical symptoms due to his mental agitation in face of a problem he misconceives as insoluble, and by utilizing these symptoms for the purpose of securing his retreat.

It is very obvious that we are influenced not by 'facts' but by our interpretation of facts. The greater or lesser sureness with which we interpret actual facts depends upon experience, which is always inadequate, upon the fact that our interpretations are not contradicted, and upon the success with which our actions correspond with our interpretations. This is especially true of inexperienced children and of asocial adults. It is easy to understand that these criteria are frequently insufficient for this purpose, since the sphere of our activity is often limited, and also since minor mistakes and contradictions are often more or less smoothly adjusted either without any effort or with the help of other persons. This assists us in keeping permanently to our life-pattern once it has been formed. It is only the more flagrant mistakes that compel us to give them closer consideration, and even this proves effective only in the case of persons who take part in the social solution of life's problems and are not pursuing any goal of personal superiority.

Thus we reach the conclusion that every one possesses

an 'idea' about himself and the problems of life—a life-pattern, a law of movement—that keeps fast hold of him without his understanding it, without his being able to give any account of it. This law of movement arises within the narrow compass of childhood. It develops by utilizing freely, and without much discriminating selection, innate powers and the influences of the external world; nor is this process restricted by any action that can be mathematically formulated. It is the artistic work of the child to direct and use for his own purpose all 'instincts' and 'impulses', as well as the impressions received from the external world and from education. This cannot be taken in the sense of 'psychology of possession' (*Besitz*), but of the 'psychology of use' (*Gebrauch*). Types, similarities, approximate likenesses are often either merely entities that owe their existence to our poverty of speech (which is incapable of giving simple expression to nuances that are always present), or they are events of a statistical probability. The evidence of their existence should never be allowed to degenerate into the setting up of a fixed rule; it can never bring us any nearer to the understanding of the individual case; it can only be used to throw light on a field of vision in which the individual case in its uniqueness has to be found. The diagnosing of an acute feeling of inferiority, for instance, tells us nothing as yet of the nature and characteristics of the individual case, nor does it give proof of any defects in education or in the social environment. These defects manifest themselves in ever-varying form in the attitude of the indivi-

27

dual to the outside world. This form is different for each individual, because of the intervention of the creative power of the child and of his interpretation springing from it.

Some schematic examples may explain what has just been said. A child who has suffered since birth from gastro-intestinal trouble, i.e. from some congenital inferiority of the digestive apparatus, but who does not receive an entirely appropriate diet—and this is nearly always the case—will in this way be led to take an exaggerated interest in food and in everything connected with it.[1] His ideas of himself and of life are thereby bound up more closely with an interest in nutrition. Later on this interest may also be directed towards money, owing to the connection between food and money that is soon perceived, but this must certainly be proved afresh in each separate case.

A child whose mother from his earliest years has relieved him of all effort, i.e. a spoilt child, will seldom be inclined even in later life to look after his affairs himself. When we compare this with parallel phenomena we are entitled to say that the child lives in the belief that everything ought to be done for him by other persons. Here, too, as well as in the following cases, only far-reaching verifications can give us the requisite certainty of judgement. We may conjecture that a child who in his early years has been given the opportunity of imposing his will on his parents will throughout his

[1] cf. Adler, *Studie über Minderwertigkeit von Organen und ihre seelische Kompensation* (Hirzel, Leipzig, 2nd edition).

28

life invariably want to dominate other persons, and in most cases the result is that the child, after experiences of an opposite kind, adopts a 'hesitant attitude' to the external world[1] and draws back into the family with all his fantasies—sexual fantasies often included—without making the necessary adjustment in accordance with social feeling. A child who in his early years has been brought up in the way best suited to his capacities as a co-worker, in the widest sense of the word entitled to equal rights, will always strive to solve all his life problems in accordance with his conception of the right social life, so long as no superhuman demands are made upon him.[2]

In the same way a girl whose father is unfair to her and neglects his family can easily come to believe that all men are like him. This is more likely to happen if she has similar experiences with a brother, with relatives, or with neighbours, or comes across them in her reading. In such a case, after the preconceived belief has been held for a short time, other experiences of a different kind scarcely count. If a brother happens to be chosen for advanced education at a university or with a view to a profession, this can easily lead to the erroneous meaning that girls are either incapable or are unjustly excluded from a higher education. If one of the children in a family feels himself kept in the background

[1] cf. Adler, *Praxis und Theorie der Individualpsychologie* (Bergmann, Munich, 4th edition).

[2] The fact that even students of Individual Psychology of many years' standing 'mean' in this connection present-day communities and not one *sub specie aeternitatis* shows that the standard of Individual Psychology is too high for them.

29

and neglected, he may become possessed with a feeling of being intimidated, as though he wanted to say: 'I shall always have to stay in the background.' Or, owing to his having the belief that he, too, is capable of achievement he will struggle furiously to surpass every one and will allow no one else to count. A mother who pampers her son excessively can instil into him the idea that simply for his own sake he must always be in the centre of things without playing a real part himself. If she nags him and criticizes him continually, if, perhaps, she also shows pretty clearly her preference for another son, she can manage to make her son in after years suspicious in his dealings with all women, and this can have consequences that are quite incalculable. If a child is exposed to many accidents or illnesses he may form from that the belief that the world is full of dangers, and he will act accordingly. The same result with different nuances may take place if the attitude of the family towards the outside world is traditionally anxious and suspicious.

It is obvious that these myriad interpretations may and do come into conflict with the world of reality and its social demands. An individual's wrong idea of himself and of the demands of life sooner or later clashes with harsh reality, which requires solutions in accordance with social feeling. The result of this clash may be compared to an electric shock. The opinion of the unsuccessful person that his style of life cannot stand up against the demand—the exogenous factor—will not be dissolved or altered thereby. The struggle for personal superiority still continues. As a result of the shock nothing remains but a greater or less restriction to a more limited field of action, the exclusion of a task that has threatened the style of life with defeat, the retreat from the problem for which the law of movement has not supplied the right preparation. The effect of the shock, however, finds both a psychical and a physical expression. It depreciates the remainder of the social feeling and gives rise to every possible mistake in life, since it forces the individual to beat a retreat, as in the case of neurosis, or it compels him to deviate into the antisocial path. There he still uses the activity that is left him, but it by no means follows that he is acting courageously. In every case it is clear that 'interpretation' is fundamental in an individual's view of the world and determines his thinking, feeling, willing, and acting.

CHAPTER II

THE PSYCHOLOGICAL APPROACH TO THE INVESTIGATION OF THE STYLE OF LIFE

We will summarily reject no method and no way of discovering the attitude of the individual to the questions of life and of finding out the meaning which life wants to disclose to us. The individual's interpretation of the meaning of life is not a trivial matter, for it is ultimately the plumb-line of his thinking, feeling, and acting. The real meaning of life, however, is shown in the opposition that meets the individual who acts wrongly. The task of instruction, education, and healing is to bridge the distance between the real meaning of life and the erroneous action of the individual. Our knowledge of man as an individual has existed from time immemorial. To give only a single instance, the historical and personal narratives of ancient peoples—the Bible, Homer, Plutarch, and all the Greek and Roman poets, sagas, fairy-tales, fables, and myths—show a brilliant understanding of the human personality. Until more recent times it was chiefly the poets who best succeeded in getting the clue to a person's style of life. Their ability to show the individual living, acting, and dying as an *indivisible* whole in closest connection with the problems of his environment rouses our admiration to the highest pitch. There can be no doubt that there were also unknown men of the people who were in advance of others in their knowledge of human nature and who passed on their experiences to their descendants. Plainly, both these men and the great geniuses in the knowledge of humanity were distinguished by their more profound insight into the connection of the mainsprings of human action with one another. This talent could only have sprung from their sympathetic bond with the community and from their interest in mankind. Their wider experience, their better knowledge, their more profound insight, came as the reward of their social feeling. There was one feature of their work that could not be missed: that was their ability to describe the myriad, incalculable expressive movements of the individual in such a way that others were able to comprehend them without needing to have recourse to weighing and measuring. This power was due to their gift of divination. Only by guessing did they come to see what lies behind and between the expressive movements, namely, the individual's law of movement. Many people call this gift 'intuition', and believe that it is the special possession only of the loftiest spirits. As a matter of fact, it is the most universal of all human gifts. Every one makes use of it constantly in the chaos of life, before the abysmal uncertainty of the future.

Since all our problems, the least as well as the greatest, are always new and always modified, we would constantly be involved in fresh mistakes if we were forced to solve them by one single method—for instance, by 'conditioned reflexes'. This perpetual variety in our problems imposes on us ever fresh demands, and forces us to test anew any mode of conduct we may have adopted hitherto. Even in a game of cards 'conditioned reflexes' are not of much use. Correct guessing is the first step towards the mastery of our problems. But this correct guessing is the specially distinctive mark of the man who is a partner, a fellow man, and is interested in the successful solution of all human problems. Peculiar to him is the view into the future of all human happenings, and this attracts him whether he is examining human history in general or the fortunes of a single individual.

Psychology remained a harmless art until philosophy took charge of it. A scientific knowledge of human nature has its roots in psychology and in the anthropology of the philosophers. In the manifold attempts to bring all human events under a comprehensive, universal law the individual man could not be disregarded. The knowledge of the unity of all the individual's expressive forms became an irrefutable truth. The transference to human nature of the laws governing every event resulted in the adoption of varied points of view, and the unfathomable, unknown regulating force was sought for by Kant, Schelling, Hegel, Schopenhauer, Hartmann, Nietzsche, and others in some unconscious motive power that was called either moral law, will, will to power, or the 'unconscious'. Along with the transference of general laws to human activity introspection came into vogue

34

By this human beings were to be able to predicate something about psychical events and the processes connected with them. This method did not remain long in use. It fell rightly into discredit because there could be no assurance of obtaining objective reports from any one.

In an age of technical development the experimental method was extensively used. With the help of apparatus and carefully selected questions, tests were arranged that were meant to throw light on the functions of the senses, on the intelligence, character, and personality. By this method knowledge of the continuity of the personality was lost, or could only be restored by guessing. The doctrine of heredity which later on came to the fore gave up the whole attempt and contented itself with showing that the main thing was the possession of capacities and not the use made of them. The theory of the influence of the endocrine glands also pointed in the same direction, and concentrated on special cases of feelings of inferiority, and their compensation in the event of organic inferiority.

Psychology underwent a renaissance with the advent of psycho-analysis. This resurrected the omnipotent Ruler of human destiny in the form of the sexual libido and conscientiously depicted in the unconscious the pains of hell, and original sin in the 'sense of guilt'. Heaven was left out of account, but this omission was afterwards rectified by the creation of the 'ideal-ego', which found support in Individual Psychology's 'ideal' goal of perfection. Still, it was a notable attempt to read between the lines of consciousness—a step forward towards the re-discovery of the style of life—of the individual's line of movement—and of the meaning of life, although the author of psycho-analysis, revelling in sexual metaphors, did not perceive this goal that hovers before humanity. Besides, psycho-analysis was far too cumbered by the world of spoiled children, and the result was that it always saw in this type the permanent pattern of the psychical structure, and the deeper layers of the mental life as a part of human evolution remained hidden from it. Its transitory success was due to the predisposition of the immense number of pampered persons who willingly accepted the views of psycho-analysis as rules universally applicable, and who were thereby confirmed in their own style of life. The psycho-analytic technique was directed, with great energy and patience, towards showing that expressive gestures and symptoms were connected with the sexual libido, and making human activity appear to be dependent on an inherent sadistic impulse. Individual Psychology was the first to make it sufficiently clear that these latter phenomena were artificially produced by the resentment of spoiled children. Still there is here also an approach to the recognition of the evolutionary impulse—a tentative adjustment to it. The effort is, however, unsuccessful; in the usual pessimistic fashion the idea of the death-wish is taken as the goal of fulfilment. But this is not an active adaptation; it is simply the expectation of a lingering death founded on the somewhat doubtful second basic law of physics.

Individual Psychology stands firmly on the ground of

evolution[1] and in the light of evolution regards all human striving as a struggle for perfection. The craving for life, material and spiritual, is irrevocably bound up with this struggle. So far, therefore, as our knowledge goes, every psychical expressive form presents itself as a movement that leads from a minus to a plus situation. Each individual adopts for himself at the beginning of his life, a law of movement, with comparative freedom to utilize for this his innate capacities and defects, as well as the first impressions of his environment. This law of movement is for each individual different in tempo, rhythm, and direction. The individual, perpetually comparing himself with the unattainable ideal of perfection, is always possessed and spurred on by a feeling of inferiority. We may deduce from this that every human law of movement is faulty when regarded *sub specie aeternitatis*, and seen from an imagined standpoint of absolute correctness.

Each cultural epoch forms this ideal for itself from its wealth of ideas and emotions. Thus in our day it is always to the past alone that we turn to find in the setting-up of this ideal the transient level of man's mental power, and we have the right to admire most profoundly this power that for countless ages has conceived a reliable ideal of human social life. Surely the commands, 'Thou shalt not kill' and 'Love thy neighbour', can hardly ever disappear from knowledge and feeling as the supreme court of appeal. These and other norms

[1] cf. *Studie über Minderwertigkeit von Organen* (Hirzel, Leipzig 2nd edition).

37

of human social life, which are undoubtedly the products of evolution and are as native to humanity as breathing and the upright gait, can be embodied in the conception of an ideal human community, regarded here as the impulse and the goal of evolution. They supply Individual Psychology with the plumb-line, the δὸs που στῶ, by which alone the right and wrong of all the other goals and modes of movement opposed to evolution are to be valued. It is at this point that Individual Psychology becomes a 'psychology of values', just as medical science, the promoter of evolution by its researches and discoveries, is a 'science of values'.

The sense of inferiority, the struggle to overcome, and social feeling—the foundations upon which the researches of Individual Psychology are based—are therefore essential in considering either the individual or the mass. The truth they represent may be evaded or put into different words; they may be misunderstood and attempts may be made to split hairs about them, but they can never be obliterated. In the right estimate of any personality these facts must be taken into account, and the state of the feeling of inferiority, of the struggle to overcome, and of the social feeling must be ascertained.

But just as other civilizations under the pressure of evolution drew different conclusions and followed wrong courses, so does every single individual. It is the child's work to create, in the stream of development, the mental structure of a style of life and the appropriate emotions associated with it. The child's emotional, and as yet barely grasped, capacity of action, serves him as a

38

standard of his creative power in an environment that is by no means neutral, and provides a very indifferent preparatory school for life. Building on a subjective impression, and guided often by successes or defeats that supply insufficient criteria, the child forms for himself a path, a goal, and a vision of a height lying in the future. All the methods of Individual Psychology that are meant to lead to an understanding of the personality take into account the meaning of the individual about his goal of superiority, the strength of his feeling of inferiority, and the degree of his social feeling. A closer scrutiny of the relation of these factors to one another will make it clear that they all contribute to the nature and extent of the social feeling. The examination proceeds in a way similar to that of experimental psychology, or to that of functional tests in medical cases. The only difference is that it is life itself that sets the test, and this shows how strong the bond is between the individual and the problems of life. That is to say, the individual as a complete being cannot be dragged out of his connection with life—perhaps it would be better to say, with the community. His attitude to the community is first revealed by his style of life. For that reason experimental tests, which at the best deal only with partial aspects of the individual's life, can tell us nothing about his character or even about his future achievements in the community. And even the *Gestaltpsychologie* needs to be supplemented by Individual Psychology in order to be able to form any conclusion regarding the attitude of the individual in the life-process.

39

THE PSYCHOLOGICAL APPROACH

The technique of Individual Psychology employed for the discovery of the style of life must therefore in the first place presuppose a knowledge of the problems of life and their demands on the individual. It will be evident that their solution presumes a certain degree of social feeling, a close union with life as a whole, and an ability to co-operate and mix with other persons. If this ability is lacking there can be noticed an acute feeling of inferiority in its innumerable variations together with its consequences. This in the main will take the form of evasiveness and the 'hesitant attitude'. The interrelated bodily and mental phenomena that make their appearance with it I have called an 'inferiority complex'. The unresting struggle for superiority endeavours to mask this complex by a 'superiority complex', which, ignoring social feeling, always aims at the glitter of personal conquest. Once all the phenomena occurring in a case of failure are clearly understood, the reasons for the inadequate preparation are to be sought for in early childhood. By this means we succeed in obtaining a faithful picture of the homogeneous style of life, and at the same time in estimating the extent of the divergence from social feeling in the case of a failure. This is always seen to be a lack of ability to get into contact with other people. It follows from this that the task of the educationist, the teacher, the physician, the pastor is to increase the social feeling and thereby strengthen the courage of the individual. He does this by convincing him of the real causes of his failure, by disclosing his wrong meaning—the mistaken significance he has foisted on life—and thus giving him a clearer view of the meaning that life has ordained for humanity.

This task can only be accomplished if a thorough-going knowledge of the problems of life is available, and if the too slight tincture of social feeling both in the inferiority and superiority complexes, as well as in all kinds of human errors, is understood. There is likewise required in the consultant a wide experience regarding those circumstances and situations which are likely to hinder the development of social feeling in childhood. Up till now my own experience has taught me that the most trustworthy approaches to the exploration of the personality are to be found in a comprehensive understanding of the earliest childhood memories, of the place of the child in the family sequence, and of any childish errors; in day and night dreams, and in the nature of the exogenous factor that causes the illness. All the results of such an investigation—and along with these the attitude to the doctor has also to be included—have to be assessed with great caution, and the conclusion drawn from them has constantly to be tested for its harmony with other facts that have been established.

CHAPTER III

THE TASKS OF LIFE

At this point Individual Psychology comes into contact with sociology. It is impossible to form a right estimate of an individual without knowledge of the structure of his life problems and the task they impose upon him. His essential nature is revealed to us only by his attitude towards them and by what takes place within him as the result of that attitude. We have to find out whether he plays his part, or hesitates, comes to a standstill, tries to evade his task, and seeks and invents excuses for this evasion; whether he finds a partial solution of his problem and outgrows it, or leaves it unsolved and follows courses that are injurious to the community in order to win the glory of a personal superiority.

For a long time now I have been convinced that all the questions of life can be subordinated to the three major problems—the problems of communal life, of work, and of love. As can be easily seen these are no casual questions, but confront us continually, compelling and challenging us, without allowing us any way of escape. For the answer we give to these three questions, by virtue of our style of life, is seen in our-whole attitude towards them. Since they are very closely connected with one another—and indeed because all three require for their proper solution an adequate amount of social feeling—it is easy to understand that every one's style of life is reflected more or less clearly in his attitude to all of them. This attitude is *less clear* with reference to the problem that meanwhile lies at a distance from him or offers favourable circumstances; it is *clearer* when the individual's own resources are put to a more exacting test. Problems like art and religion, which transcend the average solution, share in all three. These three arise from the inseparable bond that of necessity links men together for association, for the provision of livelihood, and for the care of offspring. They are problems with which our existence on earth confronts us. Human beings as products of this earth could subsist and develop in their cosmic relationship only by union with the community, by making both material and spiritual provision for it, by sharing in its work, by industry, and by providing for the propagation of the species. In their evolution they have been physically and mentally equipped for this by their struggle for a better bodily endowment and a better mental development. All experiences, traditions, commands, and laws were attempts, right or wrong, lasting or transient, made by humanity in its struggle to overcome the difficulties of life. The stage—certainly a very inadequate one—that has been reached up till now in this struggle is seen in our present-day civilization. The movement of the single individual, as well as of the mass, is marked by the attainment of a plus from a minus situation, and this gives us the right to speak of a permanent feeling of inferiority both in the case of the individual and of the mass: There can be no arrest of the stream of evolution. The goal of perfection draws us on.

If, however, these three problems with their communal basis of social interest are unavoidable, then it is clear that they can be solved only by persons who possess an adequate amount of social feeling. One may venture to assert that up to the present day every single individual has been capable of acquiring this amount of social feeling, but that the evolution of humanity has not advanced far enough yet for men to assimilate it so completely that it works as automatically as breathing or the upright gait. I do not doubt but that one day—perhaps far distant—this stage will be reached, unless humanity is frustrated in this development, and in our time some slight reason exists for suspecting that this may happen.

All other questions have for their object the solution of these three main problems. The subsidiary questions may be concerned with friendship, comradeship, interest in state and country, in the race, and in humanity; with good breeding, with the acceptance of the civilized functions of organs, with preparation for co-operation in sport, at school, and in teaching; with the respect and esteem that are due to the other sex, with the physical and mental training required to meet all these problems, as well as with the choice of a partner of the other sex. This preparation, whether it be right or wrong, starts from the first day of the child's life with the mother, who through the evolutionary development of mother-love is by nature the partner best suited to give the child experience of living with his fellow beings. From the mother, standing as the first fellow creature at the gateway that opens on the development of social feeling, come the earliest impulses urging the child to make his appearance in life as a part of the whole and to seek the right contact with other persons in his world.

Difficulties may arise from two quarters. On the part of the mother, if she makes contact with other persons difficult for the child by her tactless, clumsy, ignorant handling, or if she takes her task too lightly and carelessly. Or, as happens most frequently, if she makes it unnecessary for the child to help others or co-operate with them, if she smothers her child with caresses and endearments, constantly acts, thinks, and speaks for him, crippling every possibility of development and accustoming the child to an imaginary and altogether different world, where everything is done for the pampered child by other people. A very brief space of time is sufficient to lead the child to regard himself as the centre of events and to feel that all other situations and persons are hostile to him. Moreover the manifold nature of the results that are due to the child's unfettered judgement and the co-operation of his free creative power is not to be undervalued. The child uses external influences to mould them to his own mind. When a mother is too indulgent the child refuses to allow his social feeling to extend to other persons; he tries to withdraw himself from his father and his brothers and sisters, as well as from other people who do not meet him with an equal degree of affection. In forming this style of life, in adopting a meaning about life implying that everything will be easy to attain from the very first, but only by the help of others, the child in later years becomes unfitted for the solution of life's problems. He has not been prepared with the social feeling which these problems demand, and when he is confronted with them he experiences a shock which prevents him, temporarily in mild cases, permanently in the more severe, from finding a solution. The pampered child thinks it right that his mother should attend to him on every possible occasion. This goal of superiority, which he has chosen, he attains most easily by opposing the development of his functions. This opposition may be due to defiance—a temperamental disposition, which despite the explanation given by Individual Psychology, has been described by Charlotte Bühler as a stage of natural development—or it may be the result of want of interest; and this must be always understood as want of *social* interest. Other desperate attempts at explaining childish errors like retention of faeces and bed-wetting by deriving them from the sexual libido or from sadistic urges, and the belief that in this way more primitive or even deeper layers of the psychical life have been disclosed, put the cart before the horse, since they have misunderstood the fundamental disposition of children like these, namely their inordinate craving for affection. They are also mistaken in regarding the evolutionary function of organs

THE TASKS OF LIFE

as if it had always to be acquired anew. The development of these functions is just as natural a law and as natural an acquisition for humanity as speech and the upright way of walking. In the child's imaginary world these organic functions, as well as the prohibition of incest, can be evaded. This evasion is an indication of the wish to be pampered and has for its object either the exploitation of other persons or revenge and accusation, in cases where the pampering has been withheld.

Pampered children also reject in a thousand different ways any alteration of a situation that gratifies their wishes. If the change does take place, one can always observe the resistant actions and reactions by which the child either in a more active or more passive way attains his end. Whether it be a question of advance or retreat, the fully developed attitude for the most part depends on the child's degree of activity, although the external situation (the exogenous factor) demanding a solution must also be taken into account. In similar cases the successes that have been experienced furnish the model which is followed in later years. These are fobbed off as regression by many authors who have not rightly comprehended them. Some writers go still further with their conjectures. Although the psychical complex must now be accepted as an established and permanent evolutionary acquisition they attempt to trace it back to a residue from primeval times. In this way they manage to discover the most fantastic likenesses. Most of these authors are led astray by the fact that the forms of human expression—especially when the poverty of our

THE TASKS OF LIFE

speech is taken into account—resemble one another in
every age. It is merely a question of discovering another
resemblance when the attempt is made to relate all
modes of human action to sexuality.

I have made it clear that spoiled children, when they
are outside the pampered circle, feel themselves constantly threatened and act as though they were in a
hostile country. All their various traits of character—
above all their often inconceivable self-love and self-
admiration—have to harmonize with their meaning of
life. It follows clearly from this that all these traits are
artificial products, that they are acquired and not innate.
It is not difficult to understand, in opposition to the view
of so-called 'characterologists', that all character traits
signify social relationships and spring from the style of
life the child has created. Thus the long-standing dispute
as to whether man is good or evil by nature is settled.
The growing, irresistible evolutionary advance of social
feeling warrants us in assuming that the existence of
humanity is inseparably bound up with 'goodness'. Anything that seems to contradict this is to be considered as
a failure in evolution; it can be traced back to mistakes
that have been made—just as in the vast experiments of
nature there has always been material in the bodies of
animals that could not be used. A place will soon have to
be found in the doctrine of character for the fact that
qualities such as 'brave, virtuous, lazy, malevolent, stead-
fast, etc', are always the result of adjustments or maladjustments to an ever-changing external world and that
without this external world they simply could not exist.

As I have shown, there are still other handicaps in childhood which, like pampering, hinder the growth of social feeling. In our consideration of these hindrances we have once more to rule out of account any fundamental, governing, causal principle; we see in their effects only a misleading impulse that can be expressed in terms of statistical probability. Further, the variety and uniqueness of each individual manifestation should not be overlooked. Such manifestation is the expression of the well-nigh arbitrary creative power of the child in the formation of his law of movement. These other handicaps are the neglect of the child and his possession of inferior organs. Both of these deflect the child's outlook and interest away from 'living together' as pampering does, and turn his attention to his own dangers and his own welfare. Later on clearer proof will be given that security in the matter both of danger and welfare is attainable only if there is a sufficient amount of social feeling. But it can be easily understood that the conditions of our terrestrial existence are hostile to the person whose contact with them is imperfect, or who is not in harmony with them.

It can be said of all the three handicaps of childhood that the creative power of the child meets with varying success in the effort to overcome them. All success or failure depends on the style of life, on the individual's attitude to his life, and this is for the most part unknown to him. Just as we spoke of statistical probability determining the consequences of these three handicaps, so we have now to prove that the problems of life also, the great as well as small, exhibit a single but important statistical probability. That is the shock they produce which tests the individual attitude towards them. One can no doubt predict with some certainty what the consequences will be for an individual when he comes into contact with the problems of life; but we must always remember that no hypothesis can be assumed to be correct until the results have confirmed it.

The fact that Individual Psychology, unlike any other psychological method, is able by virtue of its experience and its laws of probability to divine the past is surely a strong proof of its scientific basis.

We have now to examine also those apparently subordinate problems and discover whether they too require for their solution developed social feeling. One of the most important of these is the child's attitude to the father. The normal attitude would be an almost equal interest in father and mother. But external circumstances, the father's personality, a pampering mother or illnesses, and difficulties in organic development—the care of which devolves upon the mother—may tend to create a distance between the child and the father and thus hinder the expansion of social feeling. This distance is only increased if the father intervenes with a more rigorous régime to prevent the consequences of the mother's coddling. The mother's often quite unrealized tendency to draw the child to take her part has the same effect. If the father's pampering predominates, then the child turns to him and away from the mother. When this happens it must always be understood as *the second phase in the life of a child*, and it indicates that the mother has been the cause of a tragedy for the child. If a child remains tied to his mother as the result of over-indulgence, then he develops more or less as a parasite and looks to his mother for the satisfaction of all his wants—incidentally his sexual wants as well. This takes place all the more readily because the child's awakened sexual instinct finds him in a state of mind in which he has learned to deny himself nothing and continually expects from his mother the satisfaction of all his desires. Freud's so-called Oedipus complex, which seems to him to be the natural foundation of psychical development, is nothing else than *one of the many forms that appear in the life of the pampered child*, who is the helpless sport of his excited fantasies. Here we must disagree with this same author when he forces with inflexible fanaticism all the relations of a child with his mother into a scheme for which the Oedipus complex serves him as a basis. We must also reject the assumption that girls are drawn more to their father and boys to their mother, though this seems to be accepted by many authors as a plausible fact. In cases where this does happen, and is not the result of pampering, we may see some understanding on the part of the child of his future sexual role, and it is therefore intended for a much later stage in life. The child, in a playful manner, for the most part without exercising his sexual instinct, is preparing himself for the future in much the same way as he does in other games as well. If the child shows a precocious and almost untamable sexual instinct, that means without question that he is egocentric and is usually a spoiled child who cannot deny himself any wish.

The position of the child with reference to the other members of the family, when this is regarded as a problem, can also give us some idea of the degree of his capacity for making contact with other persons. The three groups of children just described will as a rule be inclined to feel that the other children in the family—especially one younger than they—hinder them and restrict their influence. The effects are varied, but in the plastic period of the child's life they leave behind so great an impression that it can be recognized as a life-long trait. This takes the form of a lasting sense of rivalry in life, a passion for domination, and in the mildest case a permanent inclination to treat the other brother or sister as a child. In this development a good deal depends on success or failure in the competitive race. But, especially in the case of a spoiled child, one will never fail to discover, along with the consequences due to the child himself, the impression produced by his being supplanted by a younger member of the family.

Another question concerns the relation of the child to illness and the attitude he resolves to take up with regard to it. The behaviour of the parents during illnesses, especially when these seem to be serious, is noticed by the child. Children's diseases like rickets, pneumonia, whooping-cough, St. Vitus's dance, scarlet fever, sick-headaches, etc., during which the child notices the anxiety incautiously shown by the parents, can not only make the ailment seem worse than it really is, but create an unwonted habit of coddling, and give the child an immense feeling of importance without any co-operation on his part; they can also lead to a tendency towards being ill and complaining. If the unaccustomed pampering ceases on the recovery of health, the child often becomes refractory, or has a lasting feeling of ill health and complains about being tired and about want of appetite, or he coughs continually for no apparent reason. These symptoms are often regarded—in many cases wrongly—as the sequelae of illness. Children such as these are inclined to cling to the memory of their illnesses throughout their whole life. In this way they express their meaning that they are entitled to be indulged or that they have the right to plead extenuating circumstances. In such cases it should not be overlooked that, as a result of imperfect contact with external circumstances, occasion is given for a permanent increase of the sphere of feeling—a heightening of emotions and affects.

In addition to the question of the child's making himself useful at home, taking a proper part in games, or acting in a comradely manner, his entrance into a kindergarten or his going to school means a further test of his capacity for co-operation. There his ability to work with others can be observed. The degree of his excitement, the manner in which he shows his disinclination to go to school, his aloofness, his lack of interest and concentration, and a hundred other actions detrimental to schooling, such as being late, attempting to cause dis-

THE TASKS OF LIFE

turbances, an inclination to play truant, constantly losing his books and pencils, and dawdling instead of doing homework—all these symptoms indicate an imperfect training for co-operation. The psychical process in such cases is inadequately described if it is not understood that these children, whether they know it or not, are harbouring an acute feeling of inferiority. This comes to light as an inferiority complex corresponding to the description just given, in the form of shyness and agitation along with every possible bodily or mental symptom, or it appears as an egotistic superiority complex, in quarrelsomeness, in being spoil-sports, in a want of comradeship, etc. There is no suggestion of courage in this complex. Even arrogant children prove to be cowardly when it is a question of their doing useful work. Untruthfulness shows that they are on the way to underhand dealing, thieving propensities make their appearance as compensations that are due to them for their feeling of deprivation, while at the same time they are injurious to other people. No improvement results from their continual comparing and measuring themselves with abler children, but rather a gradual blunting of their faculties, and often as well as this the end of all success at school. Plainly the school in its effect is like a test, and shows from the very first day the child's capacity for co-operation. Plainly, too, the school is the proper place to increase the child's social feeling by judicious handling, so that he does not leave as an enemy of society. It was the realization of these facts that induced me to establish in the schools Advisory Boards for Individual Psychology, which help the teacher to find the proper methods of educating backward children.

There can be no question that success at school also depends chiefly on the child's social feeling; indeed, it is his social feeling shown in the school that gives us some idea of the form his life in the community will take in later years. Questions of friendship, so important afterwards for living with other persons; comradeship, with all its concomitant traits of fidelity, reliability, and readiness for co-operative action; interest in the State, in the nation, and in humanity, are all incorporated in life at school and require to be nurtured by experts. The school has it in its power to awaken and foster the spirit of fellow feeling. If the teacher is familiar with our point of view he will also be able by a friendly conversation to bring to the child's notice his want of social feeling; he will show him the cause of this deficiency and tell him how this cause can be removed; in this way he will bring him into closer contact with society. In general talks to the children he will be able to convince them that their own future and the future of humanity depend on an increase of our social feeling, and that the great mistakes in life—war, capital punishment, race-hatred, hatred of other peoples, not to speak of neurosis, suicide, crime, drunkenness, etc.—spring from a lack of social feeling and are to be looked upon as inferiority complexes, as pernicious attempts to deal with a situation in a way that is both inadmissible and unsuitable.

The problem of sex, too, which becomes noticeable at this stage, can plunge boys and girls into confusion.

Those children, however, who have been won for co-operation are exempt from this. They are accustomed to consider themselves as part of a whole, and they will never carry about with them worrying secrets without speaking to their parents about them or seeking advice from their teacher. It is different with those who have already discovered a hostile element in their family life. These children—and, once more, especially spoilt children—are the most easily intimidated and misled by flattery. The procedure of the parents in their explanation of sexual questions follows as a matter of course from their life in common. The child ought to know as much as he wants to know, and this information should be communicated to him in such a way that the new knowledge will be rightly received and assimilated. There must be no undue delay, but on the other hand haste is unnecessary. Talk among children at school about sexual questions can scarcely be avoided. The independent child who looks to the future will reject smut and will not credit foolish statements. Instruction that will make children afraid of love and marriage is of course a great mistake, but this will be accepted only by parasitical children who have no self-confidence.

Puberty, as another of life's problems, is considered by many to be a dark mystery. At this period also one simply discovers powers that have hitherto lain dormant in the child. If the child up till then has been wanting in social feeling, his period of puberty will pass with corresponding mistakes. The child's preparation for co-operation will then only be seen more clearly. He has at his disposal a greater room for movement. He has more strength. Above all, however, he is impelled to prove, in any way that is appropriate or that attracts him, that he is no longer a child, or—less frequently— that he is still a child. If the development of his social feeling has been hampered he will show more plainly than before the unsocial results of his mistaken course of life. Many children in their craze to be reckoned as grown-up will rather adopt the errors of adults than their virtues, since that course is easier for them than serving the community. Misdemeanours of all kinds will result from this. These again will be seen oftener in spoilt children than in others, because the former, accustomed to having their needs satisfied at once, always find it hard to resist temptation in any form. Girls and boys like these readily fall a victim to flattery or to the stimulation of their vanity. At this stage, too, girls are seriously menaced who have felt themselves badly slighted at home, and who can only believe that they are of any value when they hear themselves flattered.

The child hitherto in the background soon comes nearer the front in life, where he sees before him the three great problems of existence—society, work, and love. All these demand for their solution a developed interest in other persons. The preparation for this decides the issue. At this period we find unsociableness, suspicion, and malicious delight in the misfortunes of others, vanities of every description, hypersensitiveness, excitable states on meeting with other people, stage-fright, lying and fraud, slander, inordinate ambition, and many other traits. Those who have been educated for the community will make friends readily. They will also take an interest in all the problems that affect humanity and will adjust their standpoint and their behaviour to its welfare. They will not seek success by drawing attention to themselves by fair means or foul. Their life in the community will always be marked by goodwill, although they will raise their voice against persons who are dangerous to society. Even the most humane of men cannot rid themselves of a feeling of contempt.

The surface of the earth on which we live makes labour and the division of labour a necessity for humanity. Social feeling takes the imprint here of co-operative work for the benefit of others. The socially minded man can never doubt that every one is entitled to the reward of his labour, and that the exploitation of the lives and the toil of others cannot in any way further the welfare of humanity. Finally, we, the descendants of our great forefathers, who contributed to the welfare of humanity, do live after all mainly by their achievements. The great social thought expressed both in religions and in the outstanding political systems rightly demands the best possible apportioning of production and consumption. When any one manufactures shoes he makes himself useful to someone else, and he has the right to a sufficient livelihood, to all the advantages of hygiene, and to the suitable education of his children. The fact that he receives payment for this is the recognition of his usefulness in an age of developed trade. In this way he acquires a sense of his worth to society—the only possible means of mitigating the universal human feeling of inferiority. The person who performs useful work lives in a self-developing community and assists in its progress. This bond, though it is not always recognized, is so strong that it determines the general estimate of industry and laziness. Nobody would call laziness a virtue. Even the right of the man who has become workless as the result of crises and over-production, is already generally recognized at the present day. This is due to a growing social feeling, if not to the fear of a possible menace to society. Further, whatever changes the future may bring forth in the methods of the production and distribution of wealth, there will of necessity be a more adequate recognition of the power of social feeling than there is to-day, whether those changes are brought about by force or by mutual consent.

In love, so richly endowed with bodily and mental satisfactions, social feeling is seen to be the immediate and unquestionable moulder of our destiny. As in friendship and in the relationships with brothers and sisters or with parents, so in love we are concerned with a task for two persons, this time of different sex, with a view to having offspring and continuing the human species. Perhaps no other human problem is so vitally bound up with the welfare and prosperity of the individual in his social environment as that of love. A task in which two persons must be engaged has its own special form and cannot be successfully performed if it is treated as a task for one person alone. It is as though, for the right solution of the problem of love, each of these two persons has to forget his or her own self entirely and give complete devotion to the other; it is as though one life had to be formed from two human beings. To a certain degree we also come across the same necessity in friendship and in activities like dancing and sport, or in work where two persons make use of the same instrument for the same purpose. It is undoubtedly involved in this relationship that questions of inequality, mutual suspicion, hostile thoughts or feeling must be excluded from it. Moreover, it is of the very essence of love that physical attraction should not be lacking. Undoubtedly, too, it is due to the nature of evolution and its effect on the individual that physical attraction influences the choice of partners in a manner corresponding to the stage of advance that has been achieved by humanity.

Thus evolution puts our aesthetic sense at the disposal of the development of humanity by foreshadowing for us consciously or unconsciously a higher ideal in our life-partner. In addition to the obvious fact of equality in love—still so frequently misunderstood in our day both by husband and wife—the feeling of mutual devotion must also be taken into acount. This feeling of devotion is extremely often misunderstood by men, still oftener by girls, as a slavish subordination, and, especially when it is combined with the adoption of the principle of egotistic superiority in the style of life, it deters them from love or makes them incapable of fulfilling its functions. Deficiency in all these three directions—in preparation for a task requiring two persons for its performance, in the consciousness of equal worth, and in the capacity for devotion to another—characterizes all who lack social feeling. The difficulty they experience in this task misleads them into making perpetual attempts to find relief in dealing with the problems of love and marriage—the latter in the form of monogamy, which is undoubtedly the best active evolutionary adaptation. The structure of love just described, being the task and not the end of a development, demands in addition a decision final for eternity, since it is bound to have unending results in the children and in the welfare of humanity. It is a dismal prospect to realize that our mistakes and blunders, our lack of social feeling in love, can lead to our exclusion from everlasting existence on this earth in our children and in our cultural achievements. Such trifling with love as is seen in promiscuity, in prostitution, in perversions, or in the hidden retreat of the cults of nudism, would deprive love of all its grandeur and glory and all its aesthetic charm. The refusal to enter into a lasting union sows doubt and mistrust between the two partners in a common task and makes them incapable of devoting themselves entirely to one another. Similar difficulties, though varying for each individual, can be shown to be a sign of impaired social feeling in all cases of unhappy love and marriage, or of a refusal to perform functions that are justly expected. In such cases only the correction of the style of life can bring any improvement. Nor have I any doubt that trifling with love, i.e. a lack of social feeling, in promiscuity for example, has given an opening to the inroad of sexual diseases and in this way has led to the extermination of families and races. Since no rule for life has been ound to be absolutely invariable there are reasons for discussing the dissolution of the tie of love or marriage. Certainly not every one can be trusted to pronounce a right judgement for himself. For that reason this question should be dealt with by experienced psychologists who can be relied upon to give a decision in accordance with social feeling. The question, too, of birth-control has caused a good deal of commotion in our day. Since humanity has fulfilled the command to multiply and is as innumerable as the sand on the seashore, man's social feeling has no doubt become less rigorous in its demand for unlimited offspring. Besides the enormous development of technical equipment makes far too many hands superfluous. The need for co-workers has notably diminished. Social circumstances offer no inducement for further rapid propagation. The greatly enhanced standard of fitness for love is concerned more than in former days with the welfare and the health of the mother. Our growing civilization, too, has removed the boundaries that limited the creative powers and the intellectual interests of women. The technical advance of the present day allows both men and women to devote more time to culture, recreation, and amusement, as well as to the education of their children—an extension of leisure time which will be increased in the near future and, if properly employed, will in a large measure benefit both the individual himself and his dependents. All these facts have helped to assign to love, in addition to its task of providing for the propagation of the species, an almost independent part—a higher level, an enhancement of pleasure—which certainly contributes to the welfare of hu manity. This evolutionary advance,which has been gained once and for all and is moreover the mark that distinguishes man from beast, cannot possibly be checked by laws and regulation. The questions of deciding the number of children had best be left entirely to the woman, after careful consultation. In the case of arti- ficial interference with pregnancy both mother and child would probably be best safeguarded if in addition to consulting a physician a qualified psychological advi- ser were called in. He would dismiss any unwarranted reasons adduced for abortion, and if the reasons were sound he would give his permission. In a serious case the abortion could be carried out without expense in some institution.

For the right choice of a partner, however, in addition to physical and intellectual suitability and attraction the following qualities, which indicate a sufficient de- gree of social feeling, ought principally to be taken into consideration: (1) capacity for retaining friendship; (2) an ability to be interested in work; (3) more interest in the partner than in self.

Certainly the fear of having children can also be due to a thoroughly selfish motive. In whatever form this is expressed, in the last resort it can always be traced to a lack of social feeling. Such is the case when a spoilt girl simply goes on playing the pampered child in her mar- riage, or, thinking only of her personal appearance, fears and exaggerates the disfigurement of pregnancy or child-bearing. This also happens if the wife wishes to remain without a rival, and occasionally if she has entered into a loveless marriage. In many cases the 'masculine protest' plays a disastrous part in the performance of wifely functions and in the refusal of child-bearing. This attitude on the part of the woman, of protest against her sexual role, which I was the first to describe by the name I have given above, frequently gives rise to menstrual troubles and functional disorders in the sexual sphere. It always springs from a sexual role which has already been regarded in the family as subordinate. But it is essentially encouraged by our imperfect civilization, which strives both secretly and openly to assign an inferior position to women. Thus the occasion of menstruation may also in many cases lead to all sorts of troubles as a result of the girl's psychical self-defence and may reveal an imperfect preparation for co-operation. The 'masculine protest' in its varied forms, one of which appears as a passion to play the part of a man and can lead to Lesbian love, is accordingly to be regarded as a superiority complex based on the inferiority complex—'only a girl'.

In the period which belongs to love other forms of withdrawal from social interest also come into view at the same time as an imperfect preparation for vocation and for society. The worst form is undoubtedly to be seen in the youthful error of an almost complete self-seclusion from the claims of the community. As Kretschmer has discovered, this psychical ailment is closely connected with organic inferiority. His proofs supplement my discovery of the significance of organic handicaps at the beginning of life, although this author has not taken into account, as Individual Psychology has done, the importance of such organic inferiority for the construction of the style of life. The decline into neurosis under the ceaseless pressure of external circumstances that demand preparation for co-operation becomes more and more frequent. There is an increase, too, in suicide as the perfect retreat from the demands of life, and at the same time the thorough condemnation of them with a more or less spiteful intention. Dipsomania as a trick by which a man may evade social demands in an unsocial manner, as well as the morphia and cocaine habit, are temptations which persons without social feeling, in their flight from the problems of society, can withstand only with difficulty when these problems confront them with increased demands. Any one who has had sufficient experience in the treatment of persons such as these can prove again and again that they have a strong desire for pampering and for ease in life. The same holds good for a large number of delinquents, in whom the lack of social feeling in the activity which they exercise and at the same time their want of courage are already clearly in evidence in their childhood. One need not be surprised if at this period perversions also become more manifest. These are for the most part regarded by the perverts themselves as the result of heredity. Thus the symptoms of perversion in childhood are considered by them and by many authors as well to have been innate or contracted as the result of some experience. As a

E 65

THE TASKS OF LIFE

matter of fact they prove to be traces of a misdirected
training, and at the same time they are always a clear
sign of a defective social feeling, which comes to light
plainly enough in other aspects of their nature.[1]

Further tests of the degree of social feeling are given
in marital relationships and in the management of a
business; on the loss of a loved one, when the bereaved
person gives up the whole world as lost, although he
has never taken any part in it before; on the loss of
property, on experiencing disappointments of any kind,
where the pampered person shows himself incapable in
trying circumstances of keeping in unison with the whole
community. Many, too, on the loss of a situation, instead
of trying to combine with the community, for the purpose of removing the adverse conditions by common
action, are plunged into confusion and are forced to act
in an antisocial manner.

I will mention one last test—the fear of growing old
and the fear of death. These will not terrify the person
who is certain of his immortality in the form of his children and in the consciousness of his having contributed
to the growth of civilization. Very frequently, however,
the fear of complete annihilation is clearly evidenced in
a rapid physical deterioration and in shattered nerves.
Women are extremely often thrown into the utmost per-
plexity by the superstition of the dangerous climacteric.
Those especially who hold that the worth of women
consists in their youth and beauty and not in their power
to co-operate suffer in a remarkable way at that period.

[1] See Adler, *Das Problem der Homosexualität* (Hirzel, Leipzig).

66

They often take up, too, an attitude of defensive anta-
gonism, as though they had to meet an unjust attack,
and they fall into a state of depression which may
develop into melancholia. For me there can be no
question that the level our civilization has reached up
till now does not give elderly men and women the place
that is their due. It is their inviolable right that this
should be made possible for them, or at least that they
should have the opportunity of creating such a place
for themselves. Unfortunately the limit of their will to
co-operate is obvious at this stage. They exaggerate
their importance; they insist that they know everything
better than other people; they harp on their restrictions.
The result is that they get in the way of other people
and help to create the very atmosphere which, perhaps
for a long time, they have always feared.

After a certain amount of experience, and after calm,
sympathetic reflection, it should become clear to every
one that we are as a matter of fact being constantly
tested by the problems of life for the degree of our social
feeling and are either accepted or rejected by them.

CHAPTER IV

THE PROBLEM OF BODY AND SOUL

There can no longer be any doubt to-day that everything we call a body shows a struggle for complete wholeness. From this point of view the atom, in general, can be compared with the living cell. Both possess latent and manifest powers which give rise either to the rounding-off and delimiting of the body or to the formation of other parts. The principal difference lies in the metabolism of the cell as opposed to the self-sufficiency of the atom. Not even the internal or external movement of cell and atom shows any fundamental difference. Electrons, too, are never in a state of quiescence, and a struggle towards this state, such as Freud postulates in his theory of the death-wish, can nowhere be found in nature. The clearest point of difference between the cell and the atom is the process of assimilation and excretion in the living cell which gives rise to growth, to the preservation of form and to the struggle for an ideal final form.[1]

If the living cell, wherever it has come from, were

[1] cf. Smuts, *Wholeness and Evolution* (Macmillan, London).

placed in an ideal environment which would have guaranteed it perpetual effortless self-preservation—certainly an inconceivable condition—then it would always remain the same. Under the stress of difficulties, which in the simplest case can be pictured as almost physical, what we somewhat vaguely describe as the life-process is of necessity forced to find some sort of relief. Varieties given in nature, and certainly existing also in numberless forms among the amoeba, bring the more favourably situated individuals nearer success and give them an opportunity of finding a better form, and along with it a better adaptation to their surroundings. In the billions of years during which life has existed on this earth there was plainly sufficient time to form human beings from the life-process of the simplest cells, and also to allow myriads of existences to perish that were unable to withstand the pressure of attacks from their environment.

According to this conception, which combines the fundamental views of Darwin and Lamarck, the 'life-process' must be regarded as a struggle which maintains its direction in the stream of evolution by aiming eternally at a goal of adaptation to the demands of the external world. Imperfect organs and functions are subjected to constant stimulation from without, and it is when such stimulation bears fruit, i.e. when the organ or function adapts itself to the outside world, that evolution takes a step forward.

This struggle towards a goal can never arrive at a peaceful end, since plainly the demands and problems set by the powers of the external world to beings created by them can never be completely satisfied. In this struggle there must also have been developed that capacity which according to the view we take of it, is called soul, spirit, psyche, reason, and includes all the other 'psychical powers'. And, although in our consideration of the psychical process we move on transcendental ground, we may assert, still keeping to our point of view, that the soul as part of the life-process and of everything included in that process must in its essential characteristic be similar to the matrix, the living cell from which it has come forth. This essential characteristic is to be found above all in the ceaseless effort to reach an advantageous settlement with the demands of the external world, to overcome death, and with that end in view to strive towards the attainment of an ideal final form, and, in common action with the bodily powers prepared for that purpose by evolution, to reach by reciprocal influence and help a goal of superiority, perfection, and security. In the development of the soul, as in the evolutionary development of the body, the direction in which the difficulties of the external world can be overcome by the correct solution of its problems is unalterably marked out. Every mistaken solution, whether it be the result of unsuitable physical or psychical development, shows its want of fitness in a defeat which can lead to the elimination and extermination of the erring individual. The defeat can extend beyond the individual and injure those associated with him—his descendants—involving families, tribes, peoples, and races in still greater difficulties. As always in evolution, these difficulties by being overcome can often lead to greater successes and to greater powers of resistance. Hecatombs of plants, animals, and human beings have, however, fallen victims to this cruel process of self-cleansing. Anything that for the present appears on the average to be able to resist has provisionally stood the test.[1] On this view it follows that in the physical process we are dealing with a struggle that has to keep the body in relation to its activities roughly in a state of equilibrium, so that it may meet victoriously the demands of the external world with their advantages and disadvantages. If only one side of these processes is kept in view we arrive at the conception of the 'wisdom of the body'.[2] But the mental process as well is compelled to depend on this wisdom, which enables it to solve successfully the problems of the external world and thus maintain a ceaselessly active equilibrium of body and mind. Within certain limits the evolutionary stage that has been reached provides for this equilibrium, while the activity is furnished by the goal of superiority found in childhood—the style of life, the law of movement of each individual.

The fundamental law of life, therefore, is that of overcoming. This is supported by the struggle for self-preservation and for bodily and mental equipoise, by bodily and mental growth, and by the striving for perfection.

In the struggle for self-preservation there are included

1 cf. Adler, *Heilen und Bilden* (Bergmann, Munich, 3rd edition) ·
2 cf. Cannon, *The Wisdom of the Body* (Norton & Co., New York)·

the understanding and avoidance of dangers, propagation as the evolutionary path to the continuation of a corporeal part beyond personal death, co-operation in the development of humanity in which the spirit of the fellow-worker is immortal, and the communal achievements of every one who has contributed to any of the goals that have been mentioned.

The miracle of evolution is manifest in the perpetual endeavour made by the body simultaneously to maintain, complete, and supplement all the parts that are vital to it. The coagulation of the blood in the case of bleeding wounds, the maintenance, to a large extent guaranteed, of water, sugar, lime, albumen, the regeneration of blood and cells, the concurrent action of the endocrine glands, are the products of evolution, and show the organism's power of resistance to external injuries. The maintenance and enhancement of this power of resistance is the result of an extensive mingling of strains, by which deficiencies can be reduced and advantages retained and augmented. Here, too, the association of men—society—has acted helpfully and successfully. The elimination of incest was accordingly scarcely anything more than a fact taken for granted in the struggle for a communal existence.

The mental equilibrium is constantly threatened. In the struggle for perfection man is always in a state of psychical agitation and feels his incapacity before the goal of perfection. It is only when he feels that he has reached a satisfying stage in his upward struggle that he has the sense of rest, of value, and of happiness. In the next moment his goal draws him farther on, so that it becomes clear *that to be a human being means the possession of a feeling of inferiority that is constantly pressing on towards its own conquest.* The paths to victory are as different in a thousand ways as the chosen goals of perfection. The stronger the feeling of inferiority that has been experienced, the more powerful is the urge to conquest, and the more violent the emotional agitation. The assault of the feelings, however—the emotions and affects—are not without their effect on the physical equilibrium. The body, through the vegetative nervous system, the vagus nerve, and the endocrine variations, undergoes a change which is shown by alterations in the circulation of the blood, in secretions, in muscular tone, and in almost all the organs. As transitory phenomena these changes are natural and only show varieties in their expression according to the style of life of the person concerned. If they persist they are called functional organic neuroses, which, like the psycho-neuroses, owe their origin to the style of life. In the case of a failure due to a fairly acute feeling of inferiority this indicates an inclination to beat a retreat from the problem confronting the individual and to secure that retreat by retaining the physical or psychical symptoms of shock that have arisen. In this way the psychical process has its effect on the body. But it also has an effect on the mind itself, since it gives rise there to all sorts of psychical failures, to omissions and commissions that are inimical to the claims of the community.

In the same manner the state of the body has its effect

on the psychical process. To judge from our experiences the style of life is formed in earliest childhood. The congenital state of the body has the very greatest influence on this. The child in his initial movements and activities experiences the validity of his bodily organs. He experiences this validity, but for a long time he has neither words nor ideas for it. Since, too, the impact of the child's environment is thoroughly different in each case, anything the child feels about his capacity for action remains permanently unknown. Employing great caution and using our experience of statistical probability, we may venture to infer from our knowledge of the inferiority of the organs—of the digestive apparatus, of the circulation of the blood, of the respiratory organs, the organs of secretion, the endocrine glands, and the organs of sense— that the child feels himself overburdened at the beginning of his life. But the manner in which he gets the better of these handicaps can only be discovered from his movements and his efforts. For in this connection the idea of causality gives us no help. Here the child's creative power is at work. Struggling within the incalculable compass of his potentialities, the child by means of trial and error receives a training and follows a broadly defined path towards a goal of perfection that appears to offer him fulfilment. Whether he struggles actively or remains passive, whether he rules or serves, whether he is sociable or egotistical, brave or cowardly, whatever be the variations in rhythm and temperament, whether he is easily moved or apathetic, the child makes his decision for his whole life and develops his law of move-

74

ment in harmony, as he supposes, with his environment. He conceives of this environment and reacts to it in his own manner. The course towards the goal differs for every individual, varying in countless details, so that only which is typical in each case can be indicated; when it comes to individual differences we are forced to take refuge in lengthy descriptions. The individual himself can scarcely give any clear account of the direction of his path without the knowledge given to him by Individual Psychology. He often describes it as the very opposite. It is a knowledge of his law of movement that first gives us the explanation. By means of this we discover its intention—the meaning of the expressive forms—be they words, thoughts, feelings or actions. How rigorously the body is subjected to this law of movement is also revealed by the trend of its functions—a form of speech usually more expressive than words, and showing the meaning more clearly than words are able to do. This form of speech is nevertheless a language of the body, and I have called it 'organ dialect'. A child, for example, who in his general behaviour is tractable, but who wets his bed at night, in that way makes his meaning clear that he is unwilling to submit to an ordered civilization. A man who pretends to be brave and who perhaps even believes in his own courage nevertheless shows by his trembling and his quickened pulse that he has lost his equipoise.

A woman thirty-two years of age complained of a violent pain around the left side of her left eye and of double vision which compelled her to keep her left eye closed. The patient had had attacks like that for eleven years; the first occurred when she became engaged to her husband. The present attack began seven months before; the pains were intermittent, but the double vision remained constant. She blamed a cold bath for her last attack and believed that her former attacks had been caused by cold draughts. A younger brother suffered from similar attacks of double vision, and her mother, too, as the result of violent headaches. In the earlier attacks the pains apparently could be felt round the right eye as well and could change from the one side to the other.

Before her marriage she had taught the violin, had also appeared at concerts, and liked her work; but she had given it up after her marriage. She was now living with her brother-in-law's family, to be nearer to the doctor, as she said, and she was quite happy there.

She described her family, especially her father, herself, and several brothers as hot-tempered and irritable. If we add to this the fact, elicited and confirmed by my questioning, that they are domineering, we find that we are dealing with a type which I have described as liable to headaches, migraine, nervous trigeminal neuralgia, and epileptiform attacks.[1]

The patient also complained of urgency of micturition that always occurred when she had any nervous strain, when she was paying calls or meeting strangers, etc.

In my work on the psychical origin of trigeminal

[1] cf. especially *Praxis und Theorie der Indivualpsychologie* (4th edition).

neuralgia I have drawn attention to the fact that in cases that are not due to organic trouble a heightened emotional tension always occurs. This makes itself clearly seen in all kinds of nervous symptoms like those noted in the case just described, and by means of vasomotor exitation; and also by the agitation of the sympathetic adrenal system at the predilection points, it can produce —most probably by changes in the blood-vessels and in the blood-supply—symptoms such as pain and even paralytic phenomena. At that time I expressed the conjecture that asymmetries of the skull, of the sides of the face, and of the veins and arteries in the head are signs which betray the likely existence of similar asymmetries in the cranium, in the meninges of the brain, and even in the brain itself; they probably affect the flow and calibre of the veins and arteries situated there. Perhaps, too, the accompanying and neighbouring nerve-fibres and cells will show a weaker development in one of the two cerebral hemispheres. Special attention should then be given to the course of the nerve-tracts; they, too, are certainly also asymmetric, and owing to the dilatation of the veins and arteries on one side may prove to be too narrow. That the emotions, especially anger, but also joy, anxiety, and grief, are able to alter the filling of the blood-vessels, can be seen in the colour of the face and, in anger, in the veins standing out on the forehead. We may assume that similar modifications are to be found in the deeper layers. Certainly many more investigations are needed to clear up all the complications that are involved.

77

If, however, in this case also we succeed in showing not only the irascibility kept on the trigger by the overbearing style of life, but also the exogenous impulse before the attack, which was more violent than any experienced up till then; if we are able to establish the permanent psychical tension existing from earliest childhood—the inferiority complex and the superiority complex, the lack of interest in other persons, self-love both in her present life and also in her memories and dreams; if, moreover, we achieve success with the treatment by Individual Psychology, and if that success is at all permanent, then further proof is thereby furnished that illnesses like nervous headaches, migraine, trigeminal neuralgia, and epileptiform attacks, in so far as they do not show organic disability, may possibly be permanently cured by a change in the style of life, by the lessening of psychical tension, and by the expansion of social feeling.

The micturition on the occasion of paying calls gives us the picture of a person far too easily excited, and shows the cause of the micturition as well as the cause of stammering and other nervous disturbances and character-traits, including stage-fright, to be exogenous and due to meeting with other persons. Here, too, the intensified feeling of inferiority is apparent. Any one with a knowledge of Individual Psychology will easily be able to perceive here the sense of dependence on other people, and, as a result of this, an increased striving for appreciation, i.e. for personal superiority. The patient herself explains that she has no special interest in other persons,

She asserts that she is not anxious and that she is able to speak to others without trouble, but she is talkative to an extraordinary degree and hardly lets me get a word in edgewise—a sure sign of a strong inclination to self-description. She is undoubtedly the ruling partner in her marriage, but she comes up against her husband's indolence and his desire for peace. He works hard, comes home tired late in the evening, and is not inclined to go out with his wife or carry on a conversation with her. If she has to play in public she suffers from violent stage-fright. The question introduced by me as an important one, What would she do if she were in good health?— a question the answer to which shows clearly the reason for the patient's timid retreat—she answers evasively with a reference to her perpetual headaches. On her left eyebrow there is a deep scar from an operation on the ethnoid sinus, an operation very soon followed by an attack of migraine. The patient persists in asserting that cold in any form hurts her and brings about all sorts of attacks. Nevertheless, before her last attack she took a cold bath, which, as she says, promptly caused the attack. The attacks are not preceded by an aura. Sickly qualms occur occasionally at the beginning of an attack, but not always. She has been thoroughly examined by several doctors, but no organic lesion has been discovered. Her cranium has been X-rayed and her blood and urine tested—with negative results. The condition of the uterus is infantile, with anteversion and anteflexion. In my *Studie über Minderwertigkeit von Organen* I have pointed out that not only are organic inferiorities

79

to be found in the case of neurotics—and the results of Kretschmer's investigations strongly confirm this—but that also in the case of organic inferiorities the sexual organs may also be expected to be in an imperfect condition. This fact was brought to light by Kyrle, who unhappily died such an early death. The case we are dealing with is an example of this.

It appeared that the patient ever since she had witnessed with the utmost horror the birth of a younger sister had had an insane anxiety about child-bearing. This confirms my warnings against bringing the facts of sex too soon to the notice of children, when it is not certain that they can understand and assimilate them. When she was eleven years old her father had accused her unjustly of having sexual intercourse with a neighbour's son. This premature contact with the sexual relationship, closely associated with terror and anxiety, made her protest against love more vigorous, and this protest appeared during her marriage as frigidity. Before entering into the marriage she asked a binding declaration from her bridegroom that he would permanently deny himself any children. Her attacks of migraine and the fear of them that constantly possessed her made it easier for her to assume a relationship that reduced conjugal intercourse to a minimum. As is often the case with ambitious girls, her love-relationships were bound to become difficult, because owing to an acute feeling of inferiority, to which our backward civilization lends support, she misunderstood them as a slight put upon women.

The feeling of inferiority and the inferiority complex —these fundamental conceptions of Individual Psychology, at one time, like the masculine protest, regarded by the psycho-analysts as a red rag by a bull—are to-day fully accepted by Freud, and are forced into his system, though only in a very much attenuated form. But this school still fails to this day to understand that a girl such as the one we have been discussing is under the continuous influence of feelings of protest which make body and mind vibrate, but only find expression as acute symptoms when there is an exogenous factor, i.e. when there is a test of the amount of social feeling present.

In this case the symptomatic signs are migraine and urgency of micturition. The chronic symptoms persisting since her marriage are fear of child-bearing and frigidity. I believe that I have to a large extent explained the migraines in the case of this irascible and overbearing person—and it appears that only persons like this, with the asymmetry described above superadded, can fall ill of migraine and similar troubles. I have still, however, to indicate the exogenous factor which gave rise to the last and extraordinarily severe attack. I cannot quite deny that in this case the cold bath brought on the attack; but I am somewhat surprised that the patient, who for such a long time well knew the harm that cold would do to her seven months previously, plunged straight away into cold water without, as she says, thinking of any risk. Was it that she had one of her angry moods? Did her attack come at that particular time because she had a convenient opportunity? Had she an opponent in

the game, such as, say, her husband, who was lovingly
devoted to her, and did she enter the cold water perhaps
like some one who wants to commit suicide out of revenge to punish a person closely attached to her? Is she
still furious against herself because she is in a rage
against another person? Does she become absorbed in
reading about migraine, consult a doctor, and try to
convince herself that she can never get well in order to
postpone the solution of her life-problems that frighten
her because of her defective social feeling?

She certainly esteems her husband highly, but she is
far from being in love with him; indeed, she has never
really been in love. When asked repeatedly what she
would do if she were permanently cured she answered
at length that she would remove to the capital, give
violin lessons there, and play in an orchestra. Any one
who has acquired the art of guessing taught by Individual Psychology would have no difficulty in understanding that this meant separation from her husband, who
was tied to the provincial town. I refer for confirmation
of this to what has been said above about her feeling so
happy in her brother-in-law's house and her reproaches
against her husband. Since her husband has a great
admiration for her and gives her incomparably the best
opportunity to ride her craving for power at full gallop,
it is naturally very difficult for her to separate from him.
I would give warning here against making the path of
separation easier in this case, and in others like it by
advice and sympathetic talk, above all against recom-
mending that a lover should be taken. Such patients

know well enough what love is, but they do not understand it, and they would not only land themselves in bitter disappointments but would put the whole responsibility for these on the doctor's shoulders, if they followed his advice. In such a case the task consists in making the woman more fit for marriage. Before this can be done, however, the mistakes in her style of life would have to be removed.

The following facts were established after a more careful examination. The left side of the face is somewhat smaller than the right. For that reason the point of the nose is slightly deflected towards the left. The left eye, the one at present giving trouble, shows a narrower opening than the right. I was unable to explain meanwhile the reason for the patient's showing the same symptoms on the right side. Perhaps she was mistaken in this.

She dreamed: 'I was at the theatre with my sister-in-law and an older sister. I said to them that they were to wait a little and I would let them see me on the stage.' Explanation: She is always seeking to show off before her relatives. She would like to play in a theatre orchestra. She thinks she is not valued sufficiently by her relatives. Here, too, the theory of organic inferiority with mental compensation which I originated, is shown to be valid. (This relationship, as ought some day to be established, lies at the basis of Kretschmer's and Jaensch's conclusions.) There can scarcely be any doubt that there is something wrong with this woman's visual apparatus. The same is true for her brother, who suffers from the same illness. I cannot decide whether it is anything more than anomalies in the blood-vessels or in the nerve-tracts. The sight is said to be normal and also the metabolism. The thyroid gland is to outward appearance unaltered. The dream about the theatre and showing herself on the stage clearly indicates a visual type that is greatly concerned with outward appearance. Her marriage and her living in the province hinder her from showing herself off. Pregnancy and a child would be a similar hindrance.

A complete cure was effected within a month. Previous to that came the explanation of the exogenous factor that had led to the last attack. She found in her husband's coat pocket a letter from a girl containing merely a few words of greeting. Her husband was able to allay her suspicion. None the less she continued to be suspicious and entertained a jealousy of her husband she had never felt before. From that time she kept watch on him. It was during this period that she took the cold bath and her attack began. One of her later dreams, following on her jealousy and her injured vanity, shows that she still keeps up her suspicions and indicates her cautious and mistrustful attitude towards her husband. She saw a cat snatch a fish and run off with it. A woman ran after the cat to recover the fish from it. The interpretation follows, without our having to make much to-do about it. She seeks in metaphorical language, in which everything sounds more emphatic, to prepare herself against a similar theft of her husband. In explanation she says that she has never been jealous, that her pride has forbidden her that vice, but that since the discovery of the letter she had considered the possibility of her husband's being unfaithful to her. When she thought of the likelihood of this her wrath increased—against the assumed dependence of the wife on the husband. Her cold bath was therefore really the revenge of her style of life for what she imagined to be the unquestionable dependence of her worth upon her husband, and for his failure to appreciate that worth. Had she not had her attack of migraine—the result of her shock— then she would have had to admit that she was worthless. This however would have been the worst that could have happened to her.

CHAPTER V

BODILY FORM, MOVEMENT, AND CHARACTER

In this chapter we shall consider the three external aspects presented by the human species—corporeal form, movement, and character—in order to estimate their value and explain their significance. A scientific knowledge of humanity must, of course, take experience as its basis. But the mere collection of facts does not give us a science. It is rather the initial step towards the formation of a science, and the collected material requires to be arranged in a reliable manner under a common principle. That a fist raised in wrath, an angry glance, loud-shouted curses, etc., are movements corresponding to an attack has become so evident a matter of common sense that the human urge to investigate and get nearer the truth—and this constitutes the essential nature of science—has no further problem in this region. Only when we succeed in bringing these and other phenomena into a wider and hitherto undiscovered relationship, in which fresh points of view open up and former problems seem to be solved or come into sight, are we justified in speaking about a science.

86

The form of human organs, as well as the external form of the human being, is more or less in harmony with the mode of living, and owes its fundamental pattern to a process of adaptation to external circumstances which has remained unaltered for long periods of time. The degree of adaptation varies in countless ways and only becomes striking in its form when a definite boundary, in some way noticeable, has been passed. A number of other factors certainly influence this basic development of the human form, and of these I shall emphasize the following.

1. The extinction of certain variants, for which there are no transitory or permanent possibilities of existence. Here there come into play not only the law of organic adaptation but also mistaken ways of existence that have overburdened larger or smaller groups (war, bad government, imperfect social adaptation, etc.). In addition to the inflexible law of heredity, more or less according to the Mendelian formula, we shall have to make allowance for the fact that organs and forms are likely to be influenced in their power of combination during the process of adaptation. The relation of the form to individual and collective handicaps can be described as a function of value.

2. Sexual selection. This, in consequence of growing civilization and of increased intercourse, seems to be working towards a uniformity of form and type, and is more or less influenced by biological and medical knowledge, as well as by the aesthetic sense which is related to this. The latter is certainly subject to changes and

mistakes. Contrasted ideals of beauty, like the athlete and the hermaphrodite, buxomness and slimness, show how these influences alter; and these alterations undoubtedly receive a notable stimulation from art.

3. The correlation of organs. Organs are related to one another as though in a secret alliance, along with the glands of internal secretion (thyroid glands, sexual glands, suprarenal glands, pituitary glands) and they are able to give one another reciprocal support or injury. So it happens that forms can exist which separately would be doomed to decay, but which in their inter-connection do not fundamentally disturb the proper and complete function of the individual. In this combined effect (*Totalitätswirkung*) the peripheral and central nervous system plays an outstanding part, because in alliance with the vegetative system it is capable of having its activities greatly enhanced, and, if properly trained physically and mentally, can add to the general functional value of the individual. For this reason even atypical and positively defective forms do not necessarily threaten the continued existence of individuals and generations, since they draw compensation from other sources of power in such a way that the individual as a whole is maintained in equilibrium and even deficiencies can be occasionally outweighed. An unbiased investigation will certainly show that the most outstanding and capable persons are not by any means to be found among the most handsome. This makes us inclined to believe that individual or race eugenics could create values only within very narrow

limits, while they would be burdened with such a vast amount of complicated factors that an error in judgement would be much more likely than an accurate result. A statistical account, however well guaranteed, could not by any means be decisive in the individual case.

The moderately short-sighted eye with its elongated formation is on the whole an undoubted advantage in our civilization. This has been organized on the basis of work done within short range, and eye-fatigue is almost entirely avoided. It is certainly a disadvantage in a right-handed civilization that forty per cent of persons should be left-handed. And yet we find among the best draughtsmen and painters and among the cleverest skilled workers a striking number of left-handed people who do masterly work with their better-trained right hands. Stout persons as well as thin are threatened with dangers that are different in kind, but more or less equal in severity, although, from the standpoint both of aesthetics and medicine, the scale seems to turn more and more in favour of slimness. A short, broad metacarpus certainly seems better suited for heavy work on account of its greater power of leverage. But technical development resulting from the perfecting of machinery renders heavy manual labour more and more superfluous. Beauty of bodily form—although we cannot deny its attraction—brings with it both advantages and disadvantages. It may possibly have struck many a one that a large number of well-formed persons are to be found among the unmarried and among those who are deprived of offspring, while less prepossessing types, because they are superior in other respects, take their part in propagating the species. How often we find in certain situations types different from those we should have expected—short-legged, flat-footed mountaineers, herculean tailors, and malformed favourites of women. In such cases only a more intimate knowledge of the psychical complications will enable us to understand these apparent contradictions. Every one has no doubt come across persons of infantile stature who are singularly mature, and masculine types who behave in an infantile manner, cowardly giants and brave dwarfs, ugly deformed gentlefolk and handsome rascals, effeminate criminals and rough-looking fellows with kindly hearts. It is a well-established fact that syphilis and dipsomania injure the seed of posterity and very frequently leave a recognizable stigma on the descendants, and it is also a fact that such posterity succumbs more easily. But exceptions are not uncommon; and only recently Bernard Shaw, still so robust in his old age, has told us about his hard-drinking father. The sway of the laws of adaptation, hard to understand because it is all too complicated, stands opposed to the transcendental principle of selection. As the poet has mourned: 'And Patroclus lies in his grave, while Thersites returns.' After the great losses in the Swedish wars there was a scarcity of men, and a law was passed compelling all who remained, the sick and maimed as well, to marry. Now, if racial comparisons can be made, the Swedes of to-day belong to the best types. Ancient Greece had recourse to the exposure of misshapen children. In the Oedipus legend we see the curse of outraged nature, or perhaps it would be better to say, of the outraged logic of human society.

Perhaps every one carries within him an ideal picture of the human form and uses it as the standard by which other persons are judged. Indeed, in life we never get beyond the necessity of guessing. Those who venture a higher intellectual flight would call it intuition. The problem that the psychiatrist and the psychologist have to face is the discovery of the norms we carry within us by which we pass judgement on the human form. Here life's experiences, often of narrow range, and the stereo-typed images to which we mostly cling in childhood, seem to decide the issue. Lavater and others have formed a system out of these. When we consider the astonishing homogeneousness of such impressions and the manner in which we picture avaricious, benevolent, evil, and criminal persons, it cannot be denied, despite all justifiable doubt, that in accordance with our hidden, well-considered standard of judgement we ask the form about its content, about its meaning. Is it the spirit that creates the body for itself?

I should like to call special attention to two works dealing with this question, because they help to throw some light on the obscure problem of form and meaning. We do not forget Carus' contributions to this subject, for the revival of which Klages deserves so much credit. Nor, among the more recent investigators, should Jaensch and Bauer be passed over. But I should like particularly to single out the notable work of Kretschmer in connection with 'bodily form and character' and my own *Study of Organic Inferiority*. The latter is much the older of the two. In that work I thought I had found traces of the connecting link leading from congenital bodily inferiority—a regular minus variant—by means of the production of a more acute feeling of inferiority, so giving rise to a special tension in the psychical apparatus. When there is a want of proper training the demands of the external world—owing to this tension—will be felt as far too hostile, and concern about the person's own ego will be heightened in a manner that is plainly egocentric. From this there will result mental hypersensitiveness, defective courage, irresolution, and an antisocial pattern of apperception. The outlook on the external world becomes an obstacle to adaptation and leads to maladjustments. Here we reach a point of view from which, using great caution and being continually on the watch for confirmations or contradictions, we can draw conclusions from the form with regard to its essential content and meaning. I must leave it undecided whether or not experienced physiognomists have instinctively followed this path beyond the boundaries of science. On the other hand I could frequently confirm the fact that the psychical training which arose from this more acute tension was able to lead to greater achievements. I believe I am not mistaken when I infer from some experience that endocrine glands, such as, for example, the sexual glands, can be improved and kept in condition by suitable psychical training and can be injured by unsuitable training. It can be no accident that I have so often found—both in the case of infantile, girlish boys and in that of hoydenish girls—a training in the reverse direction that had been set going by the parents.

Kretschmer, by contrasting the pyknoid and the schizoid types with their external differences and their special psychical processes, has made a contribution to this subject of very great value. The bridge between form and meaning lay outside his interest. His brilliant account of these facts will certainly be one of the starting points, from which we shall advance to the elucidation of our problem.

The investigator is on much firmer ground when he attacks the problem of discovering *the significance of movement*. Even here a great deal has to be left to guessing, and in every case it will be necessary to get from the facts in their whole connection with one another proofs that the conjecture has been correct. At the same time we assert herewith, what Individual Psychology always emphasized, that every movement springs from *the personality as a unity*, that in it there can be no contradictions of it, no ambivalence, no two souls. That any person can be different in the unconscious from what he is in the conscious—an artificial division, after all, that has its origin merely in psycho-analytic fanaticism—will be denied by every one who has grasped the refinements and nuances of consciousness. According as a person moves, so is his meaning of life.

Individual Psychology has attempted to give a scien-

93

tific form to the doctrine of the significance of expressive movements. Within the boundaries of this science two factors are established, which in their thousandfold variations make an interpretation of these movements possible. The one takes form in the earliest childhood and shows the urge to pass from a situation in which there is no security, to victory over it, finding a path that leads from a feeling of inferiority to one of superiority and to the release of tension. This path with its special nature and its variants has already become habitual in childhood, and it is seen as a form of movement which remains unaltered throughout the whole of life. The recognition of its particular shade of difference presupposes an artistic understanding on the part of the observer. The other factor gives us insight into the social interest of the person concerned, into the degree of his willingness or unwillingness to co-operate with his fellow men. The judgement we pass on his seeing, listening, speaking, dealing, and acting, our valuation and differentiation of all his expressive movements have in view the worth of their ability to contribute to social life. Formed in a sphere of reciprocal interest these expressive movements show at every test the degree of their preparation for contributory service. The original line of movement will always make its appearance, certainly in a thousand different forms, and it cannot disappear until death. In the unbroken course of time the urge to overcome directs every movement; and this upward-striving movement takes tone and colour from the factor of social feeling.

94

MOVEMENT, AND CHARACTER

When, now, in our search for the profoundest unities, we desire with all caution to take a step forward, we reach a viewpoint that enables us to divine how movement becomes form. The plasticity of the living form certainly has its limits, but, within these limits, movement has its own effect. In the stream of time this remains the same for generations, peoples, races. Movement becomes moulded movement—form. Thus it is possible to gain a knowledge of mankind from form, if we recognize in it the movement that shapes it.

CHAPTER VI

THE INFERIORITY COMPLEX

A long time ago I emphasized the fact that to be a
human being means to feel oneself inferior. Not every
one, perhaps, can remember that he has ever felt inferior.
Possibly, too, many may feel repelled by this expression
and would rather choose another word. I have nothing
to say against this evasion, especially as I notice that
several authors have already taken advantage of it. Some
extra-clever people imagine that they will put me in the
wrong by asserting that a child in order to have a feeling
of inferiority must before that have had a high sense of
value. The feeling of insufficiency is a positive pain, and,
at the very least, lasts as long as a task has not been
accomplished, a need relieved, or a tension released.
Plainly it is a feeling given and made possible by nature,
comparable to a painful tension that seeks relief. This relief need not necessarily be pleasurable, as Freud assumes,
but it may be accompanied by feelings of pleasure—a
conception that is in accordance with Nietzsche's position. In certain circumstances the relief of this tension
can also be accompanied by permanent or temporary

suffering, somewhat like parting from a faithless friend, or like a painful operation. Further, a painful end—which is usually preferred to pain without end—can only be appraised as pleasure by a quibbler.

Just as an infant betrays by its movements its feeling of insufficiency, its ceaseless struggle for perfection and for the solution of life's problems, so the historical movement of humanity is to be regarded as the history of its feeling of inferiority and of its efforts to find a solution of its problems. Set in motion at one time or other the material of life has been constantly bent on reaching a plus from a minus situation. It is this movement, already described by me in 1907 in my *Study of Organic Inferiority*, which we comprehend under the conception of evolution. This movement is in no wise to be regarded as leading to death; on the contrary it is directed towards achieving the mastery of the external world and does not by any means seek a compromise with it or a state of rest. When Freud asserts that men are so attracted by death that they long for it in their dreams or in other ways, this would be, even according to his conception, a premature anticipation. On the other hand there can be no doubt that there are people who prefer death to a struggle with external circumstances, because in their vanity they have an exaggerated fear of defeat. They are the people who are continually longing to be pampered, who crave personal alleviations to be provided for them by other persons.

The human body is demonstrably constructed on the principle of security. Melzer in the 'Harvard Lecture's of the years 1906 and 1907, i.e. about the same date as my own study just mentioned, has drawn attention, only in a more fundamental and comprehensive fashion, to this principle of security. If an organ has been injured another takes its place, an injured organ generates from itself restorative energy. All the organs are capable of performing more than is normally required of them; one organ suffices for several vital functions, etc. Life, for which the law of self-preservation has been ordained, has won from its biological development the energy and capacity for this purpose. The splitting-off in children and in younger generations is only a part of this safe-guarding of life.

But the ever-advancing civilization that surrounds us also points to this tendency towards a safeguard. It shows that human beings are in a permanent state of feeling their inferiority, which constantly spurs them on to further action in order to attain greater security. The pleasure and pain accompanying the struggle are only aids and rewards received on this path. A permanent adaptation, however, to present-day reality would be nothing more than an exploitation of the struggles of other persons, such as the world-picture of the spoiled child demands. The continual struggle for security urges towards the conquest of present reality in favour of a better. Human life would be impossible without this stream of civilization that carries us onwards. Man would necessarily have succumbed before the assault of the powers of nature if he had not employed them to his advantage. He lacks everything that would have made the more powerful animals his conquerors. Climatic conditions compel him to protect himself from the cold by clothes, which he takes from animals better protected than he. His organism requires artificial housing, artificial preparation of food. His life is only assured by means of division of labour and by sufficient propagation. His organs and his spirit toil continually for conquest and security. To all this have to be added his greater knowledge of life's dangers and his awareness of death. Who can seriously doubt that the human individual treated by nature in such a step-motherly fashion has been provided with the blessing of a strong feeling of inferiority that urges him towards a plus situation, towards security and conquest? And this tremendous, enforced rebellion against a tenacious feeling of inferiority is awakened afresh and repeated in every infant and little child as the fundamental fact of human development.

A child, if he is not abnormal, such as for example an idiotic child, is already subjected to the impulse of this upward development, which stimulates the growth of his body and mind. He is marked out by nature for the struggle for conquest. His smallness, his weakness, the lack of self-created satisfactions, the more trivial and the more serious forms of neglect, are definite goads to the development of his powers. He creates new, and perhaps entirely original, forms of life from the pressure of his inadequate existence. His games are always directed to a future goal and are signs of his self-creative energy that can by no means be explained by conditioned reflexes. He builds continually in the void of the future, driven by the urge of his necessity to overcome. Put under the spell of the 'must' of life, he is drawn on by his constantly increasing longing for a final goal of superiority over the earthly lot that has been assigned to him, with all its unavoidable demands. And this goal that draws him on takes tone and colour from the narrow environment in which the child struggles for conquest.

I can only find a small space here for a theoretical treatment, which I published in 1912 as being fundamental, in my work *Über den nervösen Charakter*.[1]

If such a goal of conquest exists—and evolution proves that it does—then the degree of evolution that has been attained and made concrete in the child becomes material for the creation of that goal. In other words, the child's inheritance, whether it finds expression in bodily or mental possibilities, is to be taken into account only in so far as it can be and is utilized for the final goal. Anything that is found afterwards in the development has arisen from the use of inherited material and owes its completion to the child's creative power. I have myself drawn special attention to the allurements of this inherited material. I must deny, however, that it has any causal significance, because the manifold ever-changing external world demands its elastic, creative employment. The course taken towards conquest is always maintained, although the goal of conquest, as soon as it has assumed concrete form in the world-

[1] Bergmann, Munich, 4th edition.

stream, prescribes a different direction for each individual.

Inferior organs, pampering, or neglect, frequently mislead the child into setting up concrete goals of conquest, which are in contradiction to the welfare of the individual and also to the progressive development of humanity. There is, however, a sufficient number of other cases and issues to justify us in asserting, not as a matter of causal connection, but of statistical probability, that a choice of the wrong path has been the result of a mistake. And in this connection we have to remember that every evil may take on another aspect, that every one who adheres to a definite world-view exhibits a perspective in it differing from that of other persons, that every pornographic writer has his own individuality, that every neurotic makes a distinction between himself and other neurotics, just as every delinquent distinguishes between himself and others. And it is precisely in this differentiation of every individual that the child shows his own creative power, his use and exploitation of inherited possibilities and capacities.

The same holds good for the factors in the child's surrounding world and for the methods of education. The child accepts them and uses them to make his style of life concrete; he creates for himself a goal to which he inflexibly directs his course, and in accordance with which he apperceives, thinks, feels, and acts. Once the individual's movement has been firmly grasped, no power on earth can prevent one from assuming that there is a goal towards which the movement tends.

THE INFERIORITY COMPLEX

There can be no movement without a goal, and that goal can never be reached. The reason for this lies in man's primal consciousness that he can never be lord of the world. On that account he has to transpose this idea, if at any time it emerges, to the region of miracle or to the omnipotence of God.[1]

The feeling of inferiority rules the mental life and can be clearly recognized in the sense of incompleteness and unfulfilment, and in the uninterrupted struggle both of individuals and of humanity.

Every one of the countless tasks which each day brings, and which the whole of life sets before the individual, puts him in readiness for attack. His every movement proceeds from incompleteness to completion. In the year 1909, in my book *The Aggressive Impulse in Life and in Neurosis*[2] I tried to throw more light on this subject, and I came to the conclusion that this preparation for attack arises from the style of life under the compulsion of the evolutionary urge and is a part of the whole. There is no pretext for regarding it as radically evil and deriving it from an innate sadistic impulse. If the desperate attempt is made to found the mental life on instincts that have neither direction nor goal, the urge of evolution should at least not be forgotten, nor the bent of humanity towards community inherent in evolution. In view of the vast number of spoiled and disappointed human beings, one need not wonder that the

[1] Jahn und Adler, *Religion und Individualpsychologie* (Verlag Dr. Passer, Vienna).
[2] cf. *Heilen und Bilden* (Bermann, Munich, 3rd edition).

uncritical from all strata of society accept this mistaken conception of the psychical life held by pampered and therefore bitterly disappointed people.

The child's first creative act, therefore, to which in the use of his capacities he is urged by his feeling of inferiority, is his adjustment to the circumstances of his original environment. This adjustment, different in every case, is movement, which is ultimately conceived by us as form—frozen movement—a form of life that seems to offer a goal of security and conquest. The limits within which this development takes place are those of humanity in general, and these are prescribed by the stage that has been reached in the evolution of society and of the individual. Not every life-form, however, makes proper use of this evolutionary stage, and therefore it sets itself in opposition to the trend of evolution. In previous chapters I showed that complete development of body and mind is best guaranteed when the individual, by struggling and working, fits himself into the frame of the ideal community for which he has to strive. Between those who, knowingly or unknowingly, adopt this standpoint and the large number of other persons who do not take it into account there yawns a gulf that cannot be bridged. The opposition between those two sections of humanity fills the world with petty squabbles and violent strifes. Those who struggle are building up, and are contributing to, the welfare of humanity. But even those who set themselves against the trend of evolution are not entirely worthless. Through their failures and errors, which are to a greater or less degree harmful, they compel the others to make more vigorous efforts. Thus they are like the spirit 'that ever wills the evil, but creates the good'. They rouse in the others a spirit of criticism and help them to gain fuller knowledge. They contribute to the *creative* feeling of inferiority.

Thus the lines along which the development both of the individual and the community is to proceed are prescribed by the degree of social feeling. A firm foothold is thereby gained for the judgement of right and wrong. There comes into view a method which offers a surprising degree of certainty when used not only for education and therapeutics, but also for judging divergences from the right path. The standard that comes thus into use is much more accurate than any that can be furnished by the experimental method. Here life itself sets the tests; every one of the individual's slightest expressive movements can be used as an indication of the direction in which he is moving and of his distance from the community. A comparison with the current methods of the psychiatry which measures the injurious symptoms, or the injury done to the community, shows to the advantage of Individual Psychology, although the former also endeavours to refine its methods under the spell of the upward striving of the community. This advantage is further seen in the fact that Individual Psychology does not condemn, but endeavours to improve; it takes the blame from the individual's shoulders and assigns it to the failures of our civilization, in whose imperfections all of us are implicated, and it demands co-operation for their removal. It is a sign of the low

104

stage of evolution that we have reached up till now that in order to accomplish this we have to consider not merely the strengthening of social feeling but its very existence. There can be no doubt that future generations will have incorporated social feeling in their lives, just as we have done with breathing, the upright gait, and the perception of continually moving light-impressions on the retina as stationary images.

Even those who do not understand the element in man's psychical life that nurtures the feeling of community or its command 'love thy neighbour'—all who are merely occupied with revealing the 'inner scoundrel' in men hiding slyly from discovery and punishment— are important fertilizers for upward-striving humanity. They show their backward state of development in bizarre exaggeration. Their feeling of inferiority seeks a purely personal compensation in the conviction of the worthlessness of every one else. What does seem to me dangerous is to misuse the idea of social feeling in this way—viz. by taking advantage of the occasional uncertainty of the path to social feeling in order to approve socially harmful ideas and ways of life, and to force them, in the name of salvation, on the present or even on future society. Thus capital punishment, war, and even the killing of opponents occasionally find adroit advocates. Moreover, these persons always drape themselves in the cloak of social feeling. What a proof this is of its omnipotence! All these obsolete conceptions are clear indications that this advocacy springs from a lack of confidence that a new and better way can be found, i.e. from an unmistakable feeling of inferiority. The history of humanity ought to have taught every one that even killing does not make any difference to the supremacy of advanced ideas, nor does it prevent the collapse of those that are moribund. So far as we can see there is only one case in which killing can be justified, and that is in self-defence, when our own life or the life of another person is in danger. No one has brought this problem more clearly under the purview of humanity than Shakespeare has done in *Hamlet*, although this has not been understood. In all the tragedies of Shakespeare, as well as in those of the Greek poets, the murderer and the criminal are hunted to death by the Furies; and that was in an age when deeds of blood more terrible than those of our day shocked the social feeling of those who were struggling for an ideal of society. They were also nearer to that ideal, and in the end they have prevailed. All the errors of the criminal show us the furthest limits to which his social feeling can reach. Those sections of humanity that struggle forward are accordingly in duty bound not only to give enlightenment and a right education, but also not to set severe tests prematurely for persons unschooled in social feeling. Nor should they regard them in any way as though they were able to perform tasks that would only be possible for those who have a developed social feeling, but not for any who are lacking in this feeling. The reason is that persons who are unprepared experience a shock when they come up against a problem that demands a heightened social feeling; and this, through the formation of an inferiority complex, gives rise to failures of all kinds. The structure of the criminal's nature shows clearly the style of life of a person who is endowed with energy but who has little use for society. He is one who since childhood has developed a conception of life that justifies him in making use of the 'contributions' of other people. It need no longer be a secret that this type is found predominantly among pampered children, less often among those that have been neglected. There are those who hold the view that crime is self-punishment and is to be traced to childish sexual perversions, and occasionally also to the Oedipus complex. It is not dificult to confute this view when we understand that the person who is greatly in love with metaphors in real life will all too easily get entangled in a network of similes and likenesses. Hamlet: 'Do you see yonder cloud that's almost in shape of a camel?' Polonius: 'By the mass, and 'tis like a camel, indeed.'

Childish errors like the retention of faeces, bed-wetting, inordinate affection for the mother, while not freeing himself from her apron strings, etc., are distinct marks of the spoilt child, whose sphere of life does not extend beyond his mother, but at the same time does not include some of the functions which it is the mother's task to superintend. If a feeling of titillation is combined with these childish errors, as, for example, in thumb-sucking or the retention of faeces—and this can certainly happen in the case of children more sensitive to tickling than others—or if there is a nascent sexual feeling in the parasitic existence of pampered children as a result of their attachment to their mother, these are complications and consequences which are a threat chiefly to spoiled children. The clinging to these childish errors, however, as well as to childish masturbation, deflects the child's interest away from the path of co-operation —which for different reasons, above all on account of pampering, has not been mastered—to the search for alleviation and exemption from communal life. In most cases this does not happen without at the same time being accompanied by an increase of 'security' in the bond between mother and child as a result of her greater watchfulness. (This is not in any respect a 'defence', as Freud in his mistaken interpretation of my idea of security regards it.) The want of social feeling and the increased feeling of inferiority, both intimately connected with one another, are clearly manifest in this phase of the child's life, for the most part allied with all the character-traits of an existence in a supposedly hostile environment; hypersensitiveness, impatience, strengthening of affects, fear of life, caution and greed—the latter in the form of an assumption that everything ought to belong to the child.

Difficult questions in life, dangers, griefs, disappointments, worries, losses especially of persons beloved, social stress of every description, are certainly always to be seen in the picture of the feeling of inferiority, mostly in the form of the universally recognizable affects and states of mind which we know as anxiety, sorrow, despair, shame, shyness, embarrassment, disgust, etc. They are seen in facial expressions and in bodily carriage. It is as though the muscular tone were thereby lost. Or there comes into view a form of movement, which is mostly to be observed as a withdrawal from the object that causes the emotion, or as a withdrawal from the sustained questioning of life. At the same time, within the sphere of the intellect there arise thoughts of retreat in the direction of the way of escape. The sphere of feeling, so far as we have any knowledge of it, reflects in its agitation, and in the form of its agitation, the fact of uncertainty and inferiority, for the purpose of strengthening the impulse to retreat. The human sense of inferiority, which is usually expended in the struggle to advance, is seen very vividly in the storms of life and clearly enough during serious tests. Different in expression in every case, it represents when all its manifestations are included the style of life of each separate person, and this comes into full and undivided operation in all the situations of life.

Even in the attempt to master the foregoing emotions, in self-control, in wrath, and even in disgust and contempt, one should not fail to see the activity of a style of life, formed under the compulsion of the goal of superiority and spurred on by the feeling of inferiority. While the first life-form, the intellectual, by clinging to the line of retreat from menacing problems can lead to neurosis, psychosis, and masochistic behaviour; in the other form, the emotional—apart from mixed forms of neurosis—there will be seen, corresponding to the style of life, such expressions of greater activity as the inclination to suicide, dipsomania, crime, or an active perversion. This greater activity, however, must not be mistaken for courage; that is to be found only among the socially progressive. It is obvious that we are concerned here with a rearrangement of the same style of life, and not with the fictitious process that Freud calls 'regression'. Because these life-forms resemble others that have existed before or have details in common with them we are not to conclude that they are identical, and the fact that each living being has at its disposal the wealth of its mental and bodily capital and nothing else is not to be looked upon as a relapse into an infantile or primitive human stage. Life demands the solution of the problems of society, and thus all human behaviour always points to the future even when it builds with material taken from the past.

It is always the want of social feeling, whatever be the name one gives it—living in fellowship, co-operation, humanity, or even the ideal-ego—which causes an insufficient preparation for all the problems of life. In the presence of a problem this imperfect preparation gives rise to the thousandfold forms that express physical and mental inferiority and insecurity. This defect, indeed, even at an earlier stage, evokes all sorts of feelings of inferiority, only they are not so clearly marked; but they assuredly find expression in character, movement, and bearing, in the mode of thought induced by the feeling of inferiority and in the deviation from the path of progress. All these forms expressive of a sense of inferiority strengthened by the want of social feeling become obvious at the moment when the problem becomes threatening, when the 'exogenous factor' emerges. This will not be absent in a case of 'typical failure', although it may not be found by every one. Typical failures are first created by the retention of the effects of a shock—an attempt to ease the oppression caused by a severe feeling of inferiority and a result of the uninterrupted struggle to pass from a minus situation. In none of these cases, however, will the advantage of social feeling be disputed, or the distinction between 'good' and 'evil' obliterated. In every case there is a 'yes' that emphasizes the pressure of social feeling, but this is invariably followed by a 'but' that possesses greater strength and prevents the necessary increase of social feeling. This 'but' in all cases, whether typical or particular, will have an individual nuance. The difficulty of a cure is in proportion to the strength of the 'but'. This finds its strongest expression in suicide and in psychosis, following on shocks, when the 'yes' almost disappears.

Character traits like anxiety, shyness, reserve, pessimism, mark a long-standing defective contact with other persons, and when they are more rigorously tested by fate, they are greatly intensified. They appear in neurosis, for example, as more or less strongly marked symptoms of illness. This applies also to the characteristically retarded movement of the person who is always in the rear, at a marked distance from the problem confronting him. This preference for the hinterland of life is notably strengthened by the individual's mode of thinking and arguing, occasionally also by compulsive thinking, or by useless feelings of guilt.[1] It can be easily understood that it is not the feelings of guilt that bring about the individual's aloofness from his problem, but that the defective inclination and preparation of the whole personality find the feelings of guilt useful for preventing his progress. Unreasonable self-condemnation on account of masturbation, for example, supplies a suitable pretext for remorse. Even the fact that every man looking back on his past would like to have many things undone serves in the case of persons like these as a satisfactory excuse for not taking their proper part.

The attempt to trace back failures like neurosis or crime to such deceptive feelings of guilt shows a misunderstanding of the seriousness of the situation. The course pursued in the case of defective social feeling always indicates in addition grave doubt in the face of a social problem. This doubt intensifies the shock, which, along with the resulting bodily changes, helps to turn the individual to other paths. These physical changes certainly put the whole body into a state of transitory or permanent disorder, but they mostly cause very marked functional derangements at those parts that have the greatest responsibility for the psychical disturbance. This may either be a result of organic inferiority or of being burdened by too much attention. The functional disturbance can be seen in the lowering of the muscular tone, or in its stimulation—in the hair standing on end, in perspiration, in disorders of the

[1] cf. Adler, *Praxis und Theorie der Individualpsychologie* (Bergmann, Munich, 4th edition).

heart, the stomach, and the bowels, in urgency of micturation, in difficulty of breathing, in constriction of the throat, in sexual excitation, or its opposite. Often similar disorders are intensified by difficult situations in the family circle. There may also be headaches, migraine, violent blushing, or pallor. Recent researches, especially those of Cannon, Marañón and others, have established the fact that the sympathetic adrenal system plays an important part in these changes, and also the cranial and pelvic parts of the vegetative system, and that these accordingly react in different ways on all kinds of emotions. This confirms our old conjecture that the functions of the endocrine glands—the thyroid, suprarenal, and sexual glands and the hypophysis—are influenced by the external world, and that in correspondence with the individual's style of life they respond to psychical impressions according to the strength with which they are subjectively experienced. This response is meant to restore the physical equilibrium, but it is made in an extreme, over-compensatory fashion when the individual is imperfectly equipped for solving the problems of life.[1]

The individual's feeling of inferiority can also be seen in the direction of his path. I have already spoken of great aloofness from the problems of life, of coming to a halt, and of detachment from a problem. There can be no question but that occasionally such a procedure may be shown to be correct and in accordance with social feeling. The fact that this can be justified is par-

[1] cf. Adler, *Studie über Minderwertigkeit von Organen.*

ticularly relevant to Individual Psychology, since that science always assigns only a modified value to rules and formulae, and considers itself bound to produce fresh proofs of their validity. One of these proofs consists in the individual's habitual behaviour in the movement just described. Another mode of procedure—other than the 'hesitant attitude'—that makes one suspect a feeling of inferiority can be observed in the complete or partial avoidance of a problem of life. This is complete in suicide, psychosis, habitual crime, and habitual perversion, and partial in dipsomania and other addictions. As a final example of a mode of movement arising from the feeling of inferiority I will instance, in addition, the marked limitation of the sphere of existence and the narrowing of the path of advance. This excludes important parts of the problems of life. Here, too, we must make an exception. This does not apply to those who, like artists and geniuses, dismiss from their minds the solution of individual aspects of life's problems for the purpose of making a larger contribution to the advance of the community.

I have long since made up my mind about the fact of the inferiority complex in all cases of typical failure. But I strove for a long time to find the solution of the most important problem that emerges here, namely, the way in which an inferiority complex arises from the feeling of inferiority, with its bodily and mental consequences, when there is a life-problem to be met. So far as my knowledge goes this problem, far from having been solved up to the present time, has been kept in the background by authors in their investigations. The solution came to me as it does in relation to all the other problems within the purview of Individual Psychology, from seeking the explanation of the part by reference to the whole and of the whole by reference to the part. The inferiority complex, that is, the persistence of the consequences of the feeling of inferiority and the retention of that feeling, finds its explanation in the relatively greater deficiency of social feeling. The same experiences, the same dreams, the same situations, and the same life-problems, if there should exist an absolute equality in them, have different effects on every person. In this connection the style of life and its content of social feeling are of decisive importance.

Occasionally we come across persons whose lack of social feeling has been unquestionably established (for proof of this I should like to rely only on experienced observers), and who no doubt show temporarily signs of the feeling of inferiority without having developed an inferiority complex; and this in many cases may mislead us and make us doubt the validity of this argument. Such persons may sometimes be found among those who possess very little social feeling, but who live in a favourable environment. Confirmation of the presence of an inferiority complex is always to be found in the previous life of the person concerned, in his conduct up to the present, in his being pampered in childhood, in the existence of inferior organs, and in the feeling of having been neglected as a child. In the treatment use will also be made of the other means employed by Individual

Psychology which are to be discussed later, viz. the understanding of the earliest memories of childhood, the experience of Individual Psychology with regard to the style of life as a whole, and the way in which this is influenced by the individual's position in the family sequence and the method of dream-interpretation. In the case of an inferiority complex the sexual conduct and development of an individual are only a part of the whole and are completely included in that complex.

CHAPTER VII

THE SUPERIORITY COMPLEX

The reader at this point will justifiably raise the question, Where, then, in the case of the inferiority complex, is the struggle for superiority to be found? For, as a matter of fact, if we do not succeed in showing that this struggle exists in the innumerable cases of the inferiority complex, then the science of Individual Psychology would have to record an inconsistency of such a kind that it would be bound to come to grief over it. To a large extent, however, this question has been already answered.

The struggle for superiority throws the individual back from the danger zone as soon as a defeat threatens him (due to his want of social feeling) and this finds expression in open or latent cowardice. The struggle for superiority has the effect either of keeping the individual in the line of retreat from the social problem or of forcing him to get round it. Inherent in the contradiction of his 'yes-but' it compels him to accept a meaning, which gives greater weight to the 'but' and holds him so strongly under its spell that he is merely or chiefly concerned with the effects of the shock. This takes place all the more readily since it is a question here of individuals without a proper social feeling who have been preoccupied from childhood with themselves, with their own pleasure and pain. Incidentally, in these cases there can be distinguished three types, whose inharmonious style of life has developed, in an especially clear manner, a particular aspect of their psychical life. The first type includes persons in whom the intellectual sphere dominates the expressive forms. The second type is marked by an exuberant growth of the emotional and instinctive life. A third type develops rather along the line of activity. Of course, a complete absence of any one of these three tendencies is never found. Every failure, therefore, will also show very distinctly the aspect of his style of life in the effect of the shock that has been retained. While in the case of the criminal or the suicide the active factor seems generally to be thrust into the foreground, some of the neuroses are marked by an emphasis on the emotional side, unless, as mostly happens in compulsion neurosis and in the psychoses, there is a stronger accentuation of the intellectual material.[1] The addict is certainly always an emotional type. But the escape from the fulfilment of one of the tasks of life imposes a burden on human society and makes it the object of exploitation. The lack of co-operation on the part of any one must be compensated for by the extra work of other persons, by the family, or by the community. When this

[1] Adler, 'Die Zwangneurose', *Zeitschrift für Individualpsychologie* (Hirzel, Leipzig, 1931).

happens a silent, uncomprehended strife against the ideal of society is carried on—an unceasing protest which does not aid the further development of social feeling, but aims at making a breach in it. Personal superiority, however, invariably stands in opposition to co-operation. And from this it can be seen that in the case of failures we are dealing with persons whose development for communal work has been retarded, and who already lack proper vision, hearing, speaking, and judgement. In place of common sense they possess a 'private intelligence' which they cleverly employ for the securing of their divergence from the right path. I have described the pampered child as a parasite constantly occupied with putting other persons under contribution for his needs. If a style of life should be formed from this, it can be understood that the majority of failures regard the contribution of other people as their own possession, whether it be a question of affection, of property, or of material and mental effort. Whatever vigorous measures or words society may employ to guard itself against these encroachments it must naturally exercise mildness and forbearance, more as a result of its inmost urge than of its knowledge, since its eternal task is not to punish or revenge mistakes, but to explain and remove them. But there is always a protest on the part of individuals unschooled in social feeling against compulsion to co-operate. This seems intolerable to them; it runs counter to their private intelligence and threatens them in their struggle for personal superiority. It is significant of the power of social feeling that every one recognizes divergences and errors of greater or less degree as abnormal and wrong; it is as though every one had to pay tribute to social feeling. Even authors with the illusion of a scientific method, and occasionally with the endowment of genius, see the artificially cultivated will to personal power under a disguise, and, regarding it as a vicious primal instinct, as super-humanity, or as a primeval sadistic impulse, they find themselves compelled to do reverence to social feeling in its ideal culmination. Even the criminal with the goal already before his eye has to scheme and seek a justification for his deed until he can pass beyond the boundary that still separates him from antisocial conduct. From the eternally fixed standpoint of ideal social feeling, every divergence from it appears as a cunning attempt aiming at the goal of a personal superiority. The escape from a defeat at the hands of society is linked for the majority of people like these with a sense of superiority. And when the fear of a defeat keeps them constantly at a distance from the body of fellow workers, they experience and enjoy their detachment from the tasks of life as an alleviation and a privilege which give them an advantage over other people. Even when they suffer, as they do, for example, in neurosis, they are held fast securely in their position of advantage, i.e. in their suffering, without knowing how the path of suffering is going to lead them to freedom from the tasks of life. The greater their suffering the less are they troubled, and all the more are they ignorant of the real significance of life. This suffering, so inseparably bound up with relief and deliverance from the problems of life, can only seem to be self-punishment to those who have not learned to see expressive forms as a part of the whole, or rather—and this is still more important—as an answer to questions put by the community. Like neurotics themselves they will look upon neurotic suffering as an independent entity.

The reader, or the opponent of my views, will find it most difficult of all to admit that obsequiousness, servility, dependence on others, laziness, and masochistic traits—clear indications of a feeling of inferiority—give rise to a sense of relief or even of privilege. Yet it is easy to understand that they are protests against an active, social solution of the problems of life. They also represent cunning attempts to avoid defeat when there is a call on their social feeling, of which, as is evident from their whole style of life, they possess too little. In that case they let a heavy task devolve on other persons, or they even dictate it, as in masochism, often against the will of others. In all cases of failures the privileged position assumed by the individual can be easily seen. For this position he now and then pays with suffering, complaints, and feelings of guilt; but he never withdraws from the place which, as a result of his want of preparation for social feeling, seems to provide him with a successful alibi when he is asked the question: 'Where wast thou, when I parcelled out the world?'

The superiority complex, as I have described it, seems most clearly marked in the bearing, the character-traits, and the ideas of a person conscious of his own superhuman gifts and capacities. It can also be seen in the exaggerated claims he makes on himself and on other persons. Disdain, vanities in connection with personal appearance, whether in the way of elegance or neglect, an unfashionable mode of attire, exaggerated masculine conduct in women or feminine behaviour in men, arrogance, exuberant emotion, snobbism, boastfulness, a tyrannical nature, nagging, a tendency to depreciation, which I have described as characteristic, inordinate hero-worship, as well as an inclination to fawn upon prominent persons or to domineer over people who are weak or ill or of diminutive stature, emphasizing one's own idiosyncrasies, misuse of valuable ideas and tendencies to depreciate other persons, etc., can direct attention to a superiority complex that may be discovered. Also heightened affects like anger, desire of revenge, grief, enthusiasm, habitually loud laughter, inattentive listening, or turning one's eyes away on meeting other people, directing the conversation to one's own self, habitual excitement over trivial happenings, point extremely often to a feeling of inferiority ending in a superiority complex. Credulous fancies, too, crediting oneself with the possession of telepathic or similar powers or of prophetic inspiration, justifiably arouse suspicion of a superiority complex. I should like to warn those who support the social idea not to use this idea as a superiority complex or thrust it thoughtlessly on every one. The same warning applies to a knowledge of the inferiority complex and the superstructure that disguises it. One is likely to make oneself suspected of both complexes if one makes too free with them prematurely, and the only result is an opposition that is often quite justified. Further in establishing facts of this kind the universal liability of humanity to error should not be forgotten. This implies that even worthy and distinguished persons may fall into the error of the superiority complex. To say nothing of the fact that, as Barbusse puts it so well, 'Even the most kind-hearted man cannot always rid himself of the feeling of contempt.' On the other hand, these trifling and therefore ungarnished traits may lead us to direct the searchlight of Individual Psychology on mistakes with regard to the great questions of life, and thus to understand and explain them. Words, phrases, and even the knowledge of established psychical mechanisms can contribute nothing to our understanding of the individual case. The same applies to our knowledge of types. They can, however, when we make use of conjecture, serve to illumine a definite field of vision in which we hope to find the uniqueness of a personality. This uniqueness we have also to explain to the patient in the consultation, always noting the amount of social feeling we have to supply.

If for the purpose of a brief review we reduce to their quintessence the leading ideas in the developmental process of humanity, we find ultimately three well-defined lines of movement which at different periods and in succession give value to all human action. After the passing of what was perhaps an idyllic period of some hundred thousand years, when as a result of obedience to the command 'Increase and multiply' productive land became too restricted, humanity created the Titan, the Hercules, or the Imperator as the ideal redeemer. Up till the present day—in hero-worship, in pugnacity and in war—we find among high and low the lasting echo of these departed days. The path that was followed then is still extolled as the best for advancing humanity. Born from the want of sufficient subsistence this muscular impulse leads logically to the oppression and extermination of the weak. The bully delights in a simple solution—if there is little food he claims it for himself. He loves a straight, clear settlement—when this turns out to his advantage. In a cross-section of our civilization this mode of thought is very prevalent. Women are almost entirely excluded from immediate participation in activities of this kind, they come into the picture only as the bearers of children, admirers, and nurses. The means of subsistence, however, have increased enormously. They are still increasing. Is not this system of undiluted power already an absurdity?

There still remains the question of provision for the future, and for the coming generation as well. A father pinches and scrapes for his children. He makes provision for later generations. If he provides for the fifth generation, he does so at the same time for the descendants of at least thirty-two persons of his own generation who have the same claim on his descendants.

Commodities perish. They can be changed into money. The value of commodities can be lent in the form of money. The ability of other persons can be bought. People can be ordered about; more than that, they may have a character stamped on them, a meaning of life instilled into them. They can be educated to honour might and money. They can have laws imposed on them which put them at the disposal of power and property.

In this sphere, too, woman does no creative work. Tradition and upbringing put barriers in her path. She can take part admiringly or she can stand aside in disappointment. She can do homage to power, or, as most often happens, she can protect herself against her own powerlessness. And here we must remember that a person in self-defence in most cases takes the wrong path.

The majority both of men and women are able to honour power and property, the women with passive admiration, the men with ambitious striving. Women are farther off than men from the attainment of these cultural ideals.

The power-and-property Philistine is now associated with the cultured Philistine in the common struggle for personal superiority. Knowledge is (also) power. Hitherto—as a general rule—the uncertainty of life has not been met in any better way than by the struggle for power. The time has now come to reflect whether this is the best and only means of safeguarding life and developing humanity. Something may be learned, too, from the structure of the life of women. For even up till the present day woman has not had a share in the power of cultured Philistinism.

And yet it is easy for both men and women to see that woman, given a preparation equivalent to that of man, could take a successful part in the power of Philistinism. The Platonic idea of the superiority of muscular power must surely have lost its meaning in the not-understood (the unconscious). How otherwise will the secret and open revolt of women (the masculine protest) be used to the advantage of mankind in general?

Finally, we all live as parasites on the immortal achievements of artists, geniuses, thinkers, investigators, discoverers. They are the real leaders of humanity. They are the motive power in the history of the world; we are the distributors. Until now power, property, and intellectual arrogance have been the dividing line between man and woman.

Hence the outcry and the numerous books about love and marriage.

The great achievements by which we live have always established themselves as contributions of the highest value to humanity. Their victory is not celebrated in pompous words, but it is enjoyed by all. Women, too, have certainly played their part in these great achievements, but power, property, and intellectual arrogance put obstacles in the way of the majority of them. Through the whole development of art the masculine note resounds. In that sphere woman is man's understudy and is therefore second-rate. This state of things will continue until woman discloses and develops the feminine element in art. This has already taken place in two branches of the arts—in acting and in dancing. In them woman can be herself; in them she has attained the climax of her achievements.

INTRODUCTORY QUOTE IN WEIHRICH MANUSCRIPT

CHAPTER VIII

TYPES OF FAILURES

I proceed now to deal very cautiously with the theory of types, since the student may very easily fall into the error of imagining that a type is something ordained and independent, and that it has as its basis anything more than a structure that is to a large extent homogeneous. If he stops at this point and believes that when he hears the word 'criminal', or 'anxiety neurosis', or 'schizophrenia', he has gained some understanding of the individual case, he not only deprives himself of the possibility of individual research, but he will also never be free from misunderstandings that will arise between him and the person whom he is treating. Perhaps the most accurate knowledge of my work in connection with the psychical life has been gained from my careful use of the theory of types. Certainly we cannot altogether avoid using it, for it enables us to generalize, to make something like a universal diagnosis, but it can give us very little idea of any particular case or of its treatment. It is best always to keep in mind that in every case of failure we have to do with symptoms—symptoms which

127

out of a definite feeling of inferiority that has to be discovered, have developed into a superiority complex on the impact of an exogenous factor that has demanded more social feeling than the individual has been able to supply from his childhood.

We shall make a beginning with 'difficult children'. One naturally speaks of this type only when it has been evident for a considerable time that a child does not take his rightful place in co-operation as a partner of equal worth. There is a lack of social feeling, although one quite rightly concludes that while there may have been a sufficient amount of this for ordinary circumstances, it not uncommonly proves to be inadequate under any abnormal strain at home or in school. This case occurs frequently and its phenomena are on the whole well known. From these phenomena we may be able to appreciate the value of the investigations of Individual Psychology; and this will prepare us for dealing with more difficult cases. An experimental, graphological test of an individual, separated for a brief period from his surroundings, may lead to gross mistakes, and in no wise justifies us in making recommendations to the person detached in this way from his environment, or seeking to bring him under any system of classification. It is clear from facts like these that the Individual Psychologist must obtain a knowledge of all possible social circumstances and grievances in order to have a correct view of the case. One may go still further and demand that the Individual Psychologist shall be equipped with a conception of his tasks—a conception

of the demands of life, a general outlook on the world
—that has for its goal the welfare of humanity.

I have proposed a classification of difficult children
which proves useful in many respects: into the more
passive children, such as the lazy, indolent, obedient but
dependent, timid, anxious, and untruthful, and children
with similar traits; and into a more *active type* such as
those who are domineering, impatient, excitable, and
inclined to affects, troublesome, cruel, boastful, liable
to run away, thievish, easily excited sexually, etc. No
hairs need be split in this connection, but attempts
should be made to ascertain as nearly as possible the
amount of activity present in each particular case. This
is all the more important, since in a case of completely
established failure nearly the same degree of mistaken
activity can be expected and observed as in childhood.
The approximately correct degree of activity—which
means courage here—will be found in children who
possess sufficient social feeling. If one tries to find this
degree of activity in the temperament, in the swiftness
or slowness of movement, one should never forget that
these expressive forms are a part of the style of life, and
will therefore appear in an altered direction if there has
been a cure. It is not surprising to find a much larger
percentage of *passive* failures of childhood among neurotics and of *active* failures among criminals. I am inclined
to ascribe it to imperfect observation, if a failure makes
its appearance in after life, where there has been no
difficulty in upbringing. Certainly, by way of exception,
favourable external circumstances may mask the emer-

gence of a childhood's failure, which will make its appearance on more rigorous testing.

Failures in childhood belonging to the sphere of medical psychology, apart from cases of brutal treatment, are almost exclusively to be found among spoiled dependent children, accompanied by a varying degree of activity. These are: bed-wetting, difficulties in eating, screaming at night, panting, constant coughing, retention of faeces, stammering, etc. These symptoms appear in the form of a protest on the part of the child against being roused to independence and co-operation, and they exact support from other persons. Childish masturbation, continued for a long period in spite of its having been discovered, is also a sign of this want of social feeling. It will not be enough simply to treat the symptoms and attempt merely to uproot the error. Assured success can only be expected from a heightening of social feeling.

If the more passive errors and difficulties have already shown a neurotic trend—i.e. a strongly emphasized 'yes' with a more strongly stressed 'but'—then the retreat from the problems of life is seen more clearly in the neurosis without any evident accentuation of the superiority complex. There can always be observed a stock-still attitude behind the front line of life, an aloofness from co-operation or a craving for relief, and a search for excuses in the case of failure. The lasting sense of disappointment and the fear of fresh disappointments and defeats appear in the form of retaining the shock-symptoms, which secure that a distance shall be kept from the solution of social problems. Sometimes, as frequently happens in compulsion neurosis, the sick person goes as far as to utter a mild imprecation, which betrays his displeasure with other persons. In persecution mania the patient's sense of life's hostility is seen still more clearly, and it is shown in a way no one has noticed yet in the case of remaining at a distance from the problems of life. Thoughts, emotions, judgements, and ideas always run in the direction of the retreat; hence every one can clearly recognize that *neurosis is a creative act and not a reversion to infantile and atavistic forms*. It is also this creative act originated by the style of life—the self-made law of movement that always aims in some way or other at superiority—which in its manifold forms, again in accordance with the style of life, endeavours to put obstacles in the way of the cure, until the patient is convinced and common sense gains the upper hand. Quite often, as I have made clear, this secret goal of superiority is concealed by a half-mournful, half-consoling view of all the patient might have achieved if his unique, lofty flight had not been frustrated by a trifling obstacle, for which, in most cases other people were to blame. After some experience the consultant will always find in the past history of the failure very acute feelings of inferiority, the struggle for personal superiority, and imperfect social feeling. The retreat from the problems of life becomes complete in suicide. Activity is found in the psychical structure of the suicide, but never courage; his deed is simply an active protest against useful co-operation. The stroke that falls on him does not leave other persons unscathed. The community in its upward struggle will always itself be injured by suicide. The exogenous factors that bring about the end of a too slight amount of social feeling are those we have called the three great problems of life—society, vocation, and love. In every case it is the lack of appreciation that leads to suicide and death-wishes—a defeat experienced or feared in one of the three life-problems, occasionally preceded by a phase of depression or melancholia. In the year 1912 I had completed my investigation into this psychical illness, and I was able to establish that every genuine state of melancholia, such as threats of suicide, or suicide, represents a hostile attack on other persons resulting from a too small amount of social feeling. This contribution of Individual Psychology has smoothed the path to a better understanding of this psychosis. Like suicide, into which unfortunately this psychosis frequently develops, this is due to the substitution of an act of desperation in place of co-operation useful to the community. Loss of property, or of a situation, disappointments in love, set-backs of all kinds, can bring about, in accordance with the law of movement, this act of desperation in a form in which the sufferer does not shrink even from the sacrifice of those related to him or of other persons as well. Any one who is sharp of hearing psychologically will not fail to observe that he is dealing here with persons who are more easily disappointed with life than others, because they expect too much from it. In accordance with their style of life one

1 cf. Adler, *Praxis und Theorie der Individualpsychologie.*

132

may rightly expect to find in their childhood a high degree of susceptibility to shock combined with long-continued depression, or with a tendency to injure themselves as though for the purpose of punishing other persons. As more recent researches have established, the effect of a shock, which is far more severe for them than for the normal person, brings about physical changes as well. These may possibly be under the influence of the vegetative and endocrine systems. A more exact investigation will no doubt prove, as has been shown in most of my cases, that organic inferiority and, still more, a pampering régime in childhood, have misled the child into forming this particular style of life and have cramped the development of an adequate amount of social feeling. Quite often children such as these manifest an open or concealed inclination to break out into anger, to master all the problems, great and small, in their whole environment—to stand on their dignity.

A youth seventeen years old, the *youngest* in his family, and excessively spoiled by his mother, had to stay behind in the care of an elder sister when his mother set out on a journey. One evening, when left alone in the house by his sister, having just then to struggle with apparently insurmountable difficulties at school, he committed suicide. He left the following letter behind: 'Don't tell mother what I have done. Her present address is ——. Tell her, when she comes back, that I had no longer any enjoyment in life. Tell her to put flowers every day on my grave.'

An old woman with an incurable illness committed

suicide because her neighbour would not part with his wireless set.

The chauffeur of a wealthy man, learning on his master's death that he was not to receive the bequest that had been promised him, killed his wife and daughter and committed suicide.

A woman fifty-six years old who had been spoiled both as a child and in later years by her husband, and who also took a prominent place in society, suffered very keenly when her husband died. Her children were married and were not greatly inclined to devote themselves to their mother. She broke her femur as the result of an accident. Even after she recovered she kept aloof from society. Somehow or other she imagined that a voyage round the world would provide her with the friendly stimulus she missed at home. Two of her friends were willing to travel with her. In the larger continental cities her friends left her to herself on account of her unwillingness to move about. She fell into a state of excessive depression that grew into melancholia, and she sent for her children. Instead of them a foster-sister came and took her home. I saw this lady after three years of suffering that had shown no signs of improvement. Her chief subject of complaint was the great suffering her illness caused her children. Her family took turns in visiting her, but their feelings were dulled by the long continuance of their mother's illness, and they did not show any special interest in her. The patient was continually expressing suicidal ideas, and she never ceased to talk about the far too great solicitude shown by her family. It was evident that she received more attention than she did before her illness, and also that her appreciation of her children's care was in contradiction to her real feelings, and in particular to that devotion she expected as a pampered woman. If one puts oneself in her place it will be easy to understand how difficult it was for her to deny herself the attention for which she had paid so dearly by her illness.

Another form of activity, directed not against one's own self but against other persons, is acquired at an early stage by children who get the idea that other persons are their chattels, and who give expression to that idea by threatening the welfare, the property, the work, the health, and the life of others. To what extent they will carry their behaviour depends once more on the degree of their social feeling. And in each case this factor has again and again to be borne in mind. We can understand that this conception of the significance of life, which is expressed in thoughts, feelings, and states of mind, in character-traits and actions, but never in adequate words, can make real life with its demands for common action difficult for them. The sense of life's hostility is never absent from this attitude of always expecting an immediate satisfaction of their desires—an attitude which is felt to be entirely justified. Moreover, such a state of mind is closely bound up with the feeling of deprivation by which envy, jealousy, greed, and a striving to overcome the chosen victim, are permanently kept active at a high degree of intensity. Since the striving for useful development lags behind owing to the inadequate social feeling, and since the great expectations fostered by the mania for superiority remain unfulfilled, the heightening of affects often gives rise to attacks on other persons. The inferiority complex becomes chronic as soon as failure along the line of fellowship becomes noticeable in school, in society, or in love. Forty per cent of those who take to criminal practices are unskilled labourers who have been failures at school. A large proportion of abandoned criminals suffer from sexual disease—a sign of their imperfect solution of the problem of love. They seek their associates among those of the same kidney and demonstrate in that way the limitation of their friendly feelings. Their superiority complex springs from the conviction that they are superior to their victims, and that by carrying out their work in the right way they can snap their fingers at the laws and those who administer them. As a matter of fact, there are no criminals who do not have more to their account than can be proved against them, not to speak of the large number who have never been found out. The criminal perpetrates his deed in the illusion that he will never be caught if he carries it out properly. If he is convicted he is absolutely convinced that it was only his having overlooked some small detail that led to the detection of his crime. If we track the criminal tendency to the life of childhood, in addition to precocious activity wrongly used, with its unfriendly traits and its want of social feeling, we find organic inferiorities, pampering, and neglect as the causes that mislead an individual

136

into forming a criminal style of life. Perhaps pampering is the predominant cause. As the possibility of improving the style of life can never be excluded it is also necessary, in every individual case, to make inquiry into the degree of social feeling, and to take into account the gravity of the exogenous factor. No one is so liable to be tempted as the spoiled child who has been trained to get everything he wants. There must be an accurate knowledge of the strength of the temptation which has all the more disastrous results for the person afflicted with a criminal tendency, since he has a greater amount of activity at his disposal. Further, it is clear that in the case of the criminal we must grasp the relationship of the individual to his social circumstances. In many cases a person may have enough social feeling to keep him from committing a crime if the demands that are made on it are not too severe. This is also the explanation of the notable increase in the number of criminals when circumstances are unfavourable. But unfavourable circumstances in themselves are not the cause of crime, as is shown by the fact that in the United States there was a rise in the number of criminals at the time of the boom, when there were so many tempting opportunities of getting rich quickly and easily. No doubt in our search for the causes of a criminal tendency we come across the unpropitious milieu in which a child has lived; we find, too, a great number of criminals in certain quarters of a large city, but that by no means justifies us in concluding that the unfavourable environment is the cause of crime. It is much more obvious that in such conditions a proper

137

development of social feeling is scarcely to be expected. Besides, we should not forget that the child receives a very imperfect preparation for his after life when he grows up from his earliest years amidst deprivation and want, protesting, so to speak, against life and seeing close beside him every day the more favourable conditions in which other people live, while at the same time the development of his social feeling is in no way fostered. An excellent and very instructive illustration of this is given by Dr. Young's inquiry into the growth of crime in an immigrant religious sect. The first generation led a secluded and poverty-stricken existence, and there were no criminals. In the second generation the children were by this time attending the public schools, but were still brought up in the traditions of their sect, in poverty and piety, and already there was a fairly large number of criminals among them. In the third generation their number increased to an appalling extent.

The 'born criminal', too, is a discarded category. An erroneous conception of this kind, or the idea that crime is to be derived from a feeling of guilt, can be entertained only by those who take no account of our discoveries. These discoveries direct attention again and again to the strong feeling of inferiority in childhood, to the formation of the superiority complex, and the imperfect development of social feeling.

Many signs of organic inferiority are to be found among criminals, and in the shock-effect of being convicted there can be seen very marked metabolic changes

138

—probable indications of a constitution that finds unusual difficulty in reaching a state of equilibrium. Vast numbers of criminals have been pampered or want to be pampered, and among them there are those who were formerly neglected in their childhood. These facts will convince any one, provided the investigation is not approached with a stock phrase or a narrow formula. Organic inferiority is often very clearly seen in the ugliness of some criminals, while the suspicion of pampering receives constant confirmation from the fact that there are so many good-looking people to be found among them.

N. was one of these good-looking fellows, who was released on probation after a detention of six months. His offence was the theft of a considerable sum of money from his chief's till. In spite of the great danger of having to serve his three years' imprisonment for his next offence, after a short time he once more stole a small amount. Before the affair became known he was sent to me. He was the eldest son of a very respected family, his mother's spoiled darling. He was extremely ambitious and wanted to take the lead in everything. He chose his friends only from those who were his social inferiors and betrayed in this way his feeling of inferiority. In the earliest recollections of his childhood he was always the one who received things. In the situation which he held when he stole the larger amount, he saw round him people of very great wealth at a time when his father had lost his position and was unable to provide for his family in the way he had done before. Dreams of flying and dream-situations where he was the hero are signs of his ambitious striving and at the same time of his feeling that he was predestined to be successful. He committed the theft on a tempting opportunity with the idea of showing that he was better than his father. The second, smaller theft followed as a protest against his time of probation and against the subordinate position he now occupied. When he was in prison he dreamed on one occasion that his favourite dish had been brought to him, but he remembered in his dream that this was not possible in prison. In addition to the greed shown in this dream, there can easily be perceived as well his protest against his sentence.

As a rule less activity will be found among drug-addicts. Environment, want of right guidance, acquaintance with poisons like morphia and cocaine, either in illnesses or in the medical profession, provide opportunities for becoming a drug-addict. They will, however, only have a serious effect in situations where the sufferer is confronted by an apparently insoluble problem. As in the case of suicide there is seldom lacking a veiled attack on other persons who have to look after the victim. As I have shown, in the craving for drink a special component element of taste plays a part, just as, indeed, total abstinence is also made essentially easier by the want of a liking for alcohol. Very frequently the craving begins with an acute feeling of inferiority, if not with a developed superiority complex. In its earlier stages this is clearly marked by shyness, a liking for isolation, hypersensitiveness, impatience, irritability, and in nervous symptoms like anxiety, depression, and sexual insufficiency. Or the craving may start with a superiority complex in the form of boastfulness, a malicious critical tendency, a longing for power, etc. Excessive smoking, too, and the craving for strong, black coffee are often signs of a timid, irresolute state of mind. By means of a trick the burdensome feeling of inferiority is thrust aside for a time, or, as in criminal deeds, for example, it may even be transformed into increased activity. In all cases of drug-addiction every failure will be attributed to the unconquerable vice, whether the failure be in social relations, in work, or in love. Further, the immediate effects of the poison often give the victim a feeling of being delivered from his burden.

A man of twenty-six, born eight years after his sister, grew up under favourable circumstances to be excessively spoiled and self-willed. He remembered being often dressed up as a doll and held in the arms of his mother or his sister. At the age of four he came for two days under the sterner rule of his grandmother, and on the first words of refusal she uttered he packed his bag and wanted to return home. His father drank, and this upset his mother badly. At school his parents' influence gave him far too great an advantage over the other scholars. Just as he had done when he was four years old, he left his parents' house also when his mother's pampering diminished with the passing of time. As often happens with spoiled children, he could not gain a footing among strangers, and fell into an anxious state of depression and tension in social gatherings, in his business life,

and in dealing with girls. He managed to get on better
with another sort of people, who taught him drinking
habits. When his mother learned of this, and particularly when she heard that he had been in trouble with
the police when he was under the influence of drink,
she went to him and besought him in touching words
to give up drinking. The result was that he not only
sought further relief in drinking, but at the same time
he received from his mother the former care and pampering to a greater extent than ever.

A student, twenty-four years old, complained of constant headaches. While still at school he had shown
severe nervous symptoms of agoraphobia. He was
allowed to take his final examination at home. After
that his condition greatly improved. In the first year
of his university course he fell in love with a girl and
married her. Shortly after his marriage his headaches
began again. In the case of this extremely ambitious
and inconceivably spoiled man the cause of these headaches was his jealousy of his wife and his constant dissatisfaction with her. Evidence of this was plainly to be
found in his attitude and in his dreams, though he had
never fully realized it himself. Thus, on one occasion he
dreamed that he saw his wife dressed as though she were
going out hunting. As a child he suffered from rickets
and he remembered that his nurse, when she wished
to be free of him—he was always wanting to have
other people occupied with him—laid him on his back,
although he was four years old; he could not raise himself from this position by his own efforts because he was

so stout. As the second-born he lived in constant conflict with his elder brother, and always wanted to be first. Favourable circumstances enabled him to attain a high position for which he was qualified by his intellectual, but not by his psychical powers. In the troubles inevitably caused by his situation he took to morphia. He occasionally freed himself from the drug, but he always fell a victim to it again. Once more his unreasoning jealousy came into play to make his situation more difficult. As he felt himself insecure in his post he committed suicide.

CHAPTER IX

THE UNREAL WORLD OF THE PAMPERED

Pampered people are not in good repute. They never were. Parents are not fond of being accused of pampering. The spoiled person himself refuses to be regarded as such. Again and again a doubt occurs as to what we mean by pampering. But, as though by intuition, everyone feels it as a burden and an obstacle to proper development.

Nevertheless, every one likes to be petted. Quite a number of people show an extraordinary liking for being coddled. Many a mother can do nothing but pamper her children. Fortunately many children defend themselves so vigorously against such treatment that less damage is done than might be expected. This problem is a hard nut to crack when only using psychological formulae. We cannot use these formulae rigidly as guiding lines to be followed blindly in order to discover the basic structure of a personality or the explanation of dispositions and characters. We must rather expect to find in every direction countless variants and nuances, and we must always confirm what we think we have discovered and compare it with facts that are parallel to it. For when a child sets himself against pampering he usually carries his opposition too far and transfers his resistance to other situations where it would be reasonable to expect friendly help from the outside world.

When pampering is established in later life, without being linked, as often happens in such cases, with the crushing of free will, it may easily at times make the pampered person disgusted with it. But this will still leave unchanged the style of life that has been acquired in childhood.

Individual Psychology asserts that there can be no other way of understanding a human being than by the study of the movements he makes for the solution of his life-problems. The mode of his movements and his reasons for making them have to be carefully observed. His life starts out with the possession of human potentialities and possibilities of development that are assuredly different for every one, and it is only a person's actions that can give us a criterion for judging these differences. Everything we are able to discover at the beginning of his life is already strongly influenced by external circumstances from the day of his birth. The influences both of heredity and environment become the child's possession, and he uses them for the purpose of finding his path of development. But neither the path nor the movement can be thought of, or adopted, without a direction and a goal. *The goal of the human soul is conquest, perfection, security, superiority.*

THE UNREAL WORLD OF THE PAMPERED

The child in his employment of the influences he has experienced from his own body and from the surrounding world is more or less dependent on his own creative power and on his ability to divine a path. His interpretation of life—which is at the bottom of his attitude to life and is neither shaped into words nor expressed by ideas—is his own masterpiece. Thus the child acquires his law of movement which aids him after a certain amount of training to form his style of life, and in accordance with this we see the individual thinking, feeling, and acting throughout his whole existence. This style of life has almost always developed in a situation where the child is assured of outside support. In the ever-varying conditions of existence such a style of life does not seem to be suited to stand the test when anything that requires unselfish assistance has to be done in the world outside the home.

The question now arises as to what is the right attitude in life, and what solution of life's problems is to be expected. Individual Psychology endeavours as far as possible to answer these questions. No one is blessed with the possession of absolute truth. A concrete solution which is universally correct must be valid in two respects. A thought, a feeling, or an act is to be characterised as right only when it is right *son specie aeternitatis* (in the light of eternity). And, further, the welfare of the community must be incontestably included within it. This holds good for tradition as well as for fresh problems that arise, and it applies to the lesser problems as well as to those that are vital. The three great problems that each has to solve, and has to solve in his own fashion—the problems of society, work, and love—can be met in an approximately right way only by those in whom the struggle for the community has become a living fact. Unquestionably there will be doubt and uncertainty when fresh problems emerge; but only the existence of the will to co-operate can be a safeguard against gross mistakes.

When we come across types in our investigation we are not exempted from the duty of discovering the uniqueness of the individual case. This applies also to pampered children—that constantly increasing burden on the home, the school, and society. We have to discover the peculiarity of each case, whether we are dealing with difficult children, nervous or insane persons, suicides, delinquents, drug-addicts, or perverts, etc. They all suffer from a lack of social feeling that can almost always be traced back to pampering in childhood, or to an excessive craving for pampering and relief.

A person's active bearing can only be discovered by a correct understanding of his movement when he is confronted by the problems of life. This applies also to the lack of movement. Nothing of importance is gained for the knowledge of the individual case by attempting, like the *Besitz*-psychologists (possession-psychologists), to trace every kind of symptom of failure to the obscure regions of an uncertain heredity, or to influences from the surrounding world, universally regarded as unsuitable. The child, exercising a certain amount of freedom

147

of choice, accepts these influences, assimilating and reacting to them. Individual Psychology is a psychology of use, and it emphasizes the creative appropriation and utilization of all these influences. Any one who regards the various problems of life as unalterable, and does not perceive their uniqueness in every separate case, can easily be led to believe in efficient causes, in impulses and instincts as the demonic rulers of our destiny. No one who recognizes that problems that have never existed before emerge for every new generation can believe in the working of an inherited unconscious. Individual Psychology is too well acquainted with the groping and searching of the human spirit and with its artistic activities, be they right or wrong, in the solution of its problems, to accept that belief. It is the activity of each separate person resulting from his style of life that conditions his own solution of his problems. The value of the theory of types to a large extent disappears when the poverty of human speech is realized. How different are the relationships which we describe with the word 'love'! Are two introverted persons ever the same? Is it conceivable that the lives of two identical twins, who, by the way, very frequently wish and strive to be identical, can ever take a uniform course here beneath the changing moon? We can employ the idea of types, indeed we must employ it, just as we do the conception of probability, only we should never forget, even when we are dealing with similarities, the difference invariably shown by each separate person. In our expectation of the course a case will follow, we can make use of probability for the purpose of throwing light on the field of vision in which we hope to find the unique event, but as soon as we encounter contradictions we must deny ourselves its aid.

In our search for the roots of social feeling—presupposing the possibility of its development in man—we at once come across the mother as the first and most important leader. Nature has given her this position. Her relation to the child is that of an intimate co-operation (community in life and work) in which there is a mutual gain. It is not, as many believe, a one-sided exploitation of the mother by the child. The father, the other children in the family, relatives, and neighbours, have to further this work of co-operation by training the child to become a fellow worker of equal standing and not an antagonist of society. The more deeply the child is impressed with the reliability and the partnership of other persons the more he will be inclined for communal life and independent co-operation. He will put all he possesses at the disposal of co-operative effort.

On the other hand, whenever the mother abounds all too evidently with excessive affection and makes behaviour, thought, and action, and even speech, superfluous for the child, then he will be more readily inclined to develop as a parasite (exploiter) and look to other persons for everything he wants. He will continually press forward to be the centre of every scene and seek to have every one at his beck and call. He will display egoistic tendencies and regard it as his right to suppress other people and to be always pampered by them—to

149

take and not to give. A year or two of such training will be sufficient to put an end to the development of his social feeling and any inclination to work with other persons.

At one time dependent on other people, at another longing to suppress them, such children soon come up against the opposition, insurmountable for them, of a world that demands fellowship and co-operation. Robbed of their illusions, they blame other people and always see only the hostile principle in life. Their questions are of a pessimistic nature. They ask: 'Has life any meaning?' 'Why should I love my neighbour?' If they submit to the legitimate demand of an active social idea, it is only because they are afraid that they would be rebuffed and punished if they opposed it. Confronted with the problems of community, work, and love, they are not able to find the path of social interest; they suffer a shock and feel its effects in body and mind, and they beat a retreat either before or after they are conscious of having suffered a defeat. But they always keep to their accustomed childish attitude, which implies that a wrong has been done to them.

We can now also understand that all characteristic traits are not only not innate, but above all that they express relations entirely determined by the style of life. They are the by-products of the child's creative activity. The spoiled child, misled into self-love, will develop egoistic, envious, jealous traits in a high degree of intensity, although also of varying amount. He will live as though he were in a hostile country and will manifest hypersensitiveness, impatience, want of perseverance, a tendency to passionate outbursts, and a greedy nature. An inclination to beat a retreat and an excessive cautiousness usually accompany these traits.

The gait—to speak metaphorically—of a pampered person is not easily detected when circumstances are favourable to him. It is much easier to do this when his situation is unfavourable and he is being tested for the content of his social feeling. In such a situation he is found in a hesitant attitude, or he comes to a halt at a fairly great distance from his problem. He gives fictitious reasons for keeping this distance, and these prove that his action has not been the result of shrewdness and caution. He often changes his society, his friends, his partner in love, and his occupation without carrying anything to a successful issue. Occasionally people like these rush forward so hurriedly when they begin to do anything that the expert knows at once how little self-reliance there is to be found in such haste and how soon the zeal will cool down. Others become eccentrics who would prefer to retire to the desert in order to avoid all their problems. Or they find only a partial solution of their problem, and by doing so they greatly limit their sphere of action in a manner that corresponds to the degree of their feeling of inferiority. When they have at their disposal a certain amount of activity, which is certainly not to be called 'courage', they easily turn aside in a situation that is in any way oppressive, to join the socially useless—indeed, the socially injurious—and become criminals, suicides, drunkards, or perverts.

THE UNREAL WORLD OF THE PAMPERED

It is not easy for every one to identify himself with the life of an excessively pampered person, in other words, to understand him completely. One has to master this role like a good actor and, getting inside this whole sphere of existence, to understand how to make oneself the central figure, and how to keep a sharp look-out for every situation where one oppresses other people and never is a fellow worker, where one must expect everything and give nothing. In order to understand that people like these are not guided by reason, it is necessary to realize how they try to exploit for themselves the communal work of other persons—their friendship, their labour, and their love; how their sole interest is in their own welfare, their own personal exemption from effort, and how they never think of anything else but the easing of their own tasks to the detriment of other persons. The psychically healthy child develops courage, a reasoning power universally valid, and a capability for active adaptation. The spoiled child has none of these qualities; he has instead of them cowardliness and cunning. Withal he has an extraordinarily restricted path, and the result is that he always seems to make the same mistakes. The tyrannical child always appears tyrannical. The pickpocket always keeps to his trade. The anxiety-neurotic always reacts to all his life's tasks with anxiety. The drug-addict sticks to his poison. The sexual pervert shows no inclination to give up his perversion. In their elimination of other activities, in the narrow path along which their life has its course, there can be easily seen once more their cowardliness, their want of self-confidence, their inferiority complex, their tendency to shut themselves off.

The dream-world of pampered persons—their perspective, their meaning and grasp of life—is immensely different from the real world. Their power of adaptation to the evolution of humanity is more or less choked, and this brings them into a ceaseless conflict with life which involves other people in its harmful results. In childhood we find them both among over-active and among passive children; in later life they are to be seen among criminals, suicides, neurotics, and drug-addicts, and they are always different from one another. For the most part dissatisfied, they look with fierce envy on the success of other persons, without attempting to do anything on their own behalf. Always under the spell of a dreaded defeat, of the discovery of their worthlessness, they are mostly seen in retreat from the tasks of life—a retreat for which they are never at a loss to find excuses.

It should not be overlooked that many of them are successful in life. They are those who have conquered by learning from their mistakes.

The cure and the transformation of such persons can only be accomplished by following the path of the spirit, by the growing conviction on their part that they have failed in the construction of their style of life. Prevention is easier than cure; the family, especially the mother, must understand that love for the child should not grow into pampering. More might be expected from a body of psychologically trained teachers who have learned to recognize and correct these errors. It will then become clearer than it has appeared up till now that there is no greater evil than the pampering of children, with all its consequences.

Individual Psychology, by proving that every individual's conception of life is determined by, and is a part of, the person's style of life, has thrown light upon the rather bewildering fact that philosophers and psychologists differ widely in their interpretations of the inner world. It is plain that each of them regards mind and psyche from a viewpoint that is determined by his philosophy of life. Thus an author whose wrong conception of life is like that of a pampered child will inevitably declare that all trouble arises because the individual is unable to 'get' what he wants. And he will take it for granted that all failures, neuroses, psychoses, delinquencies, suicides, perversions are due to the fact that these people have suppressed their wishes. These authors will also find that the real world is hostile and destined to perish. Social interest is for them a mystical dogma forced upon people by illusions or fear. 'Love thy neighbour as thyself' is for them merely ridiculous. But the relationship between the individual and the mother —the pampering person—they consider to be of highest importance. Automatically they close their eyes to other conflicting views.

Authors afraid of losing ground or of being assailed by criticism, attach importance only to those facts that are capable of receiving physical confirmation in laboratories and that can be recorded and reduced to figures. They feel protected by mathematical rules and they become irritable if they are without such symbols. Of course, mathematics gives a great feeling of security and provides support for many persons. But, when we study mind and psyche, we find that they are the gifts of evolution and have been spread over millions of years. They work like miracles, and all we can discover about them is the manner in which they function in relation to outside problems. We have to keep in mind, too, that the body and its inherited qualities are simply parts of the general environment.

And Individual Psychology? Has it not also its own particular conception of life? Has it not also a specific point of view regarding the behaviour of the individual in his relation to outside problems? Of course it has. But in the first place we have tried to prove that our conception of life is more capable of objectivity than the conceptions of other psychologists. And secondly *we know* that we also are predisposed by our philosophy of life, while others do *not* know that they always find what they have known before. For this reason Individual Psychology is more capable of detachment and self-control.

Finally, Individual Psychology has another exceedingly important advantage. The Individual Psychologist recognizes that the personality is a *unity*, and thus he is compelled to see that the individual's misconception of one aspect of life will be repeated in all the others. The same lack of social interest will characterize *all* the expressive forms of an erring individual.

No psychologist is able to determine the meaning of any expression if he fails to consider it in its relation to society.

CHAPTER X

WHAT REALLY IS A NEUROSIS?

Any one who has occupied himself with this problem year in, year out, will understand that the question— What then is the real nature of a neurosis?—has to receive a clear and straightforward answer. If we explore the literature on the subject with the object of finding an explanation, we discover such a confusion of definitions that in the end a uniform conception of neurosis can scarcely be reached.

As is always the case when there are obscurities connected with any question, we find a multitude of explanations, and many opposing factions spring up. This has happened with the problem of neurosis. Neurosis is irritability, irritable weakness, disease of the endocrine glands, the result of dental or nasal infection, disease of the genital organs, weakness of the nervous system, the result of a hormonal or of a uric acid diathesis, of a birth trauma, of a conflict with the external world, with religion, with ethics, a conflict between a vicious unconscious and a consciousness inclined to compromise, of the suppression of sexual, sadistic, criminal impulses, of the noise and the dangers of a city, of a lax or of a rigorous upbringing, of an upbringing especially in the family, of certain conditioned reflexes, etc.

There is a great deal in these views that is of value and that can be utilized for the explanation of some of the more or less important phenomena that constitute a neurosis. But most of these phenomena may frequently be found in the case of persons who do not suffer from a neurosis. Only a few of them point the way to a clarification of the question—What really is a neurosis? The enormous frequency of this disease, its extraordinarily disastrous social consequences, and the fact that only a small proportion of nervous subjects undergo any treatment, but carry their illness about with them in extreme agony their whole life long; and, in addition, the great interest in the subject that has been stirred up among the laity, justify a cool, scientific elucidation of it before a larger tribunal. One can also realize that a great deal of medical knowledge is needed for the understanding and treatment of this disease. Further, we should always bear in mind the fact that the prevention of neurosis is possible and necessary, but that this can only be expected from a clearer knowledge of the injuries that have caused it. The measures to be adopted for its prevention, and for the understanding of its insignificant beginnings, belong to the sphere of medical science. But the assistance of the family, of teachers, educationists, and other helpers is indispensable. This justifies a wide diffusion of all that is known about the nature and origin of a neurosis.

Arbitrary definitions, such as have existed for a long time, must be unconditionally rejected, for example, that it is a conflict between the conscious and the unconscious. There can be little discussion on this point, for the authors who support this view must ultimately have realized that nothing at all can take place without conflict, so that this statement sheds no light on the nature of a neurosis. Nor, too, is any light to be got from those who take up a lofty scientific standpoint and want to mislead us by attributing those organic changes to chemical action. They will find it difficult to make any contribution in this way to the solving of the problem, since we can make no pronouncements about chemical action. Neither do the other current definitions tell us anything new. What is understood as a nervous state is irritability, suspicion, shyness, etc.—in short, any kind of manifestations that are marked by negative qualities, by character traits that are not suited to life and seem to be loaded with affects. All authors agree that the nervous state is connected with a life of intensified affects. When many years ago I set about describing what we understand by the nervous character I brought to light the hypersensitiveness of the nervous person. This trait is certainly to be found in every nervous subject, although in some exceptional cases it cannot be discovered very easily, since it is concealed; closer examination, however, shows that such persons are none the less acutely sensitive. Individual Psychology by its more

158

thorough research, has shown the source of this sensitiveness. Any one who feels at home on this poor earth-crust of ours, who is convinced that he has to share not only its delights but its drawbacks, and is resolved to make some contribution to social well-being, will not exhibit any undue sensitiveness. Exaggerated sensitiveness is an expression of the feeling of inferiority. From this there follow quite naturally the other traits of the nervous person, such as, for example, impatience. This, too, is not shown by the person who feels himself secure, who has self-confidence, and has reached the point of coming to terms with the problems of life. When these two character-traits of hypersensitiveness and impatience are kept in view, it will be understood that there are people who live in a state of intensified emotion. And when we add that this feeling of insecurity leads to a violent struggle for a state of repose and security, then it can be seen why the nervous person is spurred on in his striving for superiority and perfection. It can be understood too, that this trait, with its implication of a struggle for pre-eminence, takes the form of ambition —an ambition that is solely concerned with the person himself. This is intelligible in the case of a person who is in straits. Occasionally this striving for pre-eminence takes other forms, such as greediness, avarice, envy, and jealousy, which, as a matter of course, are universally condemned. Here it is a question of persons who are violently straining every nerve to outwit their difficulties, because they have no confidence in their own powers to find a straightforward solution. Add to this that the intensified feeling of inferiority goes hand in hand with an imperfect development of courage, that instead of this we find a number of cunning attempts to evade the problem of life, to make existence easier, and to throw the load on the shoulders of other persons. This evasion of responsibility is bound up with a lack of interest in other people. We are far from setting out to criticize or condemn the large number of people who to a greater or less extent show this attitude; we know that even the worst mistakes are not made with a conscious sense of responsibility, but that the person in question has become the victim of a wrong attitude towards life. These persons have before them a goal the pursuit of which brings them into conflict with reason. Still nothing has been said yet of the nature of the nervous state, of the way in which it has been brought about, or of the factors which go to its formation. We have, however, taken one step in advance, and, taking into account the defective courage of the nervous person and his hesitant attitude towards the tasks of life, we were able to show the meagre result of his life-process in face of the problems of life. It is certain that we can trace this meagre amount of activity back to the period of childhood. As Individual Psychologists we are not surprised at this, because the life-pattern is developed in the earliest years of childhood and is only accessible to change if the person in question understands the error in his development and has the power to come once more into contact with other people with a view to the welfare of humanity as a whole.

160

WHAT REALLY IS A NEUROSIS?

It may be assumed that a child who shows more than
the normal amount of activity of the wrong kind, if he
becomes a failure in after life, will never be a nervous
subject. His failure will take another form and he will
become a criminal, a suicide, or a drunkard. It is possible he may turn out to be a 'difficult' child of the worst
sort, but he will never develop the traits of a nervous
person. We have approached then a little nearer to the
solution of our problem. We can assert that the radius
of action in the case of the nervous subject does not
extend very far; it is much more restricted than that of
a more normal person. It is important to know the
source of the greater amount of activity in the other
cases. If we can prove that it is possible either to develop
or restrict a child's radius of action, if we have understood that in a wrong education there are means of
reducing this to a minimum, then we also understand
that the question of heredity does not influence us in
this direction, but that what we see is the product of
the child's creative power. The condition of the body
and the impressions of the external world are the building materials which the child uses for the construction
of his personality. The fact to be noted in connection
with the symptoms of nervous trouble is that they are
all chronic. These symptoms can be classified as physical
disturbances of certain bodily organs and as psychical
shocks—manifestations of anxiety, compulsion thoughts,
signs of depression (these seem to have a special significance), nervous headaches, compulsory blushing and
washing, and similar psychical expressive forms. They

persist for a long time; and if we do not betake ourselves to the obscure region of fantastic ideas, if we are willing to admit that their development has some meaning, and if we seek their connection with one another, we shall discover that the task which confronts the child has been too difficult for him. In this way the permanent nature of nervous symptoms seems to be established and explained. The outbreak of these symptoms is due to the reaction that follows on a certain definite task. We have made extensive investigations in order to discover in what the difficulty of solving problems consists, and Individual Psychology has permanently lit up this whole territory by establishing the fact that human beings are always confronted by problems for the solution of which a social preparation is required. The child must obtain this preparation in his earliest years, for any increase of it is only possible on this understanding. When we have undertaken the task of making it clear that such a problem actually results always in a shock, then we can speak about the effects of shock. Such shocks can be of various kinds. In some cases it may be a social problem—say, a disappointment in friendship. Which of us has never experienced this, or has not received a shock from it? But the shock is still no sign of nervous disease. It is a sign of nervous disease, and actually becomes nervous disease, only when it persists, when it develops into a chronic condition. In that case the person in question avoids suspiciously all personal intimacy and shows clearly that he is always prevented from coming into closer contact with other persons by shyness and embarrassment, and by bodily symptoms like a quickened pulse, perspiration, gastro-intestinal troubles, and urgency of micturition. This is a condition that has an unmistakable significance in the light thrown upon it by Individual Psychology. It tells us that this person has not sufficiently developed a sense of contact with other people; and it follows from this that his disillusionment has brought him to a position of isolation. We are now at closer grips with the problem, and we can give some idea of the nervous state. When, for example, some one loses money in business and feels the shock of this loss he has not yet become a nervous subject. This happens only when he remains in that state, when he feels the shock and nothing else. This can only be explained if we understand that a person in this state has not acquired a sufficient degree of co-operative ability, and that he goes forward only on condition of being successful in everything he attempts. The same holds good for the problem of love. Certainly the solution of this problem is not a trifling affair. For its solution some experience and understanding are required, and a certain sense of responsibility. If any one becomes excited and irritated on account of this problem, if after having been rejected once he makes no further advances, if all the emotions that secure his retreat from the problem in question play a part in that retreat, if he has such a conception of life that he keeps to his path of retreat —then, and not till then, is he a nervous subject. Every one feels a shock when he is under fire, but the effects of the shock will only become chronic if the person who has suffered them is not prepared for the tasks of life. In that case he will come to a standstill. We have already substantiated this complete halt when we said that there are people who are not properly prepared for the solution of every problem, who from their childhood have never been real co-workers. But there is something more than this to be said. It is suffering that we see in the nervous state, and not something that the victim enjoys. If I were to propose to any one that he should give himself headaches like those that result from confronting a problem for the solution of which he was unprepared he would not be able to do so. We must therefore reject at once all explanations which imply that a person produces his own suffering, or that he wants to be ill. Without doubt the person concerned *does* suffer, but he always prefers his present sufferings to those greater sufferings he would experience were he to appear defeated in regard to the solution of his problem. He would rather put up with these nervous sufferings than have his worthlessness disclosed. Both nerve-ridden and normal people offer the strongest opposition to the exposure of their defeats, but the neurotic carries his opposition much the furthest. If we try to imagine what is meant by hypersensitiveness, impatience, intensified emotion, and personal ambition, then we shall be able to understand that such a person, so long as he thinks himself in danger of having his worthlessness revealed, cannot be brought to take a single step forwards. What then is the mental state that results from these effects of a shock? The sufferer has not caused them; he does not want

164

them; they do exist, however, as the consequences of a psychical shock, as the result of his sense of defeat, of the fear of being unmasked in all his worthlessness. He has no real inclination to struggle against this result, nor does he understand how he is to free himself from it. He would like to have it removed; he will persist in saying: 'I should like to get well again, I want to get rid of the symptoms.' Accordingly he even goes and consults a doctor. But what he does not know is that he is still more afraid of something else—of being proved to be worthless. Somehow or other the sinister secret might come to light—the fact that he is of no value. We see now what a nervous state actually is. It is an attempt to avoid a greater evil, an attempt at all costs to keep up the appearance of being of some value, to spare no expense in the attainment of this goal, but at the same time there is also the desire to reach it without any cost at all. Unfortunately this is impossible. There is nothing else for it but to supply the person in question with a better preparation for life, to encourage him, and give him a firmer footing; and this cannot be done by driving him on, by punishing him, by being severe with him, or coercing him. One knows how many people there are who, when they have a certain amount of activity at their disposal, would rather do away with themselves than solve their problems. That is clear. We cannot therefore expect anything from coercion; a systematic preparation must be taken in hand, so that the sufferer shall feel himself secure and in a position to approach the solution of his problem. Otherwise we have a person who imagines he is standing before a deep abyss and is afraid that he is going to be pushed into it—i.e. that his worthlessness is going to be revealed.

A barrister of thirty-five complains of nervousness, constant pain in the back of his head, all sorts of troubles in the region of the stomach, dullness in his whole head, and general weakness and tiredness. In addition he is always excited and restless. He is often afraid of losing consciousness when he has to speak to strangers. At home in his parents' family circle he feels more at ease, although even there he does not find the atmosphere entirely congenial. He is convinced that these symptoms will prevent him from ever being successful.

The clinical examination gave a negative result, with the exception of a scoliosis, which along with the loss of muscular tone as a result of depression can go far to explain the occipital and spinal pains. The tiredness, it is plain, is due to his restlessness, but it is certainly also to be understood, like the sense of dullness in the head, as a partial manifestation of the depression. The troubles in the region of the stomach are more difficult to understand in the light of the general diagnosis we are employing in this case, but they may also be the expression of a predilection—the reaction of an inferior organ to a psychical irritation. In support of this view there are stomachic disorders that occurred frequently in childhood; and a similar complaint of his father's, which also had no organic defect to account for it. The patient knows, too, that occasional excitements were always followed by a loss of appetite and sometimes by vomiting.

WHAT REALLY IS A NEUROSIS?

A complaint which may perhaps be regarded as trifling helps us to understand more clearly the patient's style of life. His restlessness is a proof that he has not quite given up his struggle for 'success'. This same conclusion, although in lesser degree, is confirmed by his statement that he does not feel comfortable even at home. In a lesser degree, because his anxiety about meeting strangers, i.e. about going out into the world, cannot leave him even at home. His fear of losing consciousness, however, enables us to get a glimpse into the workings of his neurosis. He tells us, without being aware that he does so, that he artificially increases his agitation when he has to see strangers by a preconceived idea that he is going to become unconscious. Two reasons can be given for the patient's not knowing that artificially, as though with a purpose, he heightens his excitement into a state of confusion. The first reason is obvious, although it is not generally recognized. The patient, so to speak, only casts a furtive glance at his symptoms, and does not see their connection with his whole mode of behaviour. The other reason is that the inexorable retreat, the 'advance backwards'—described long ago by me[1] as the most important neurotic symptom—may not be interrupted, although in the case we are considering it is bound up with the patient's feeble attempts at pulling himself together. The agitation felt by the patient when he came up against the three life-problems—of society, occupation, and love—for which he is evidently

[1] *Über den nervösen Charakter* (J. F. Bergmann, Munich, 4th edition).

167

unprepared, affects not only his body, producing functional changes in it, but the psyche as well. (This agitation has certainly also to be verified, for up till now it
has only been conjectured with the help of a general
diagnostic, the experience of Individual Psychology and
medico-psychological intuition.) From this person's defective preparation there result functional disturbances
of body and mind. The patient, possibly taught by former experiences of minor failures, recoils in fear from
the 'exogenous factor'. He feels himself threatened by a
permanent defeat, all the more since as a spoilt child—
a fresh bit of evidence which we shall have to prove later
on—he finds his self-constituted goal of personal superiority with its lack of interest in other persons more and
more unattainable. In this state of highly intensified
emotion which is always caused by anxiety about a
decisive defeat, although anxiety in the ordinary sense
of the word does not show itself plainly, those symptoms
arise that we find in neurosis and psychosis. They
have their origin in accordance with the physical constitution, which is generally innate, and with the
psychical, which is always acquired. They are combined with one another and reciprocally influence one
another.

But have we yet arrived at a neurosis? Individual
Psychology has undoubtedly done a great deal to throw
light on the fact that a person can be well or badly
prepared for the solution of life's problems, and that
between the good preparation and the bad there exist
many thousand variants. It has done much, too, to help

us to understand that the feeling of being unable to solve these problems revealed by the exogenous factor causes manifold vibrations in body and mind. It has also shown that the defective preparation has its source in earliest childhood and can be put right neither by experiences nor by emotions, but by a better knowledge. Further, it has discovered that social feeling is the integrating factor in the style of life, and that this must be present in a decisive manner if all the problems of life are to be solved. The physical and psychical phenomena that accompany and characterize the sense of failure I have described as the inferiority complex. Without doubt the effects of a shock are greater for persons who have been badly prepared than for those who have had a better preparation, less for the courageous than for the cowardly, who are always looking for help from the outside. Every one has conflicts that cause him greater or less agitation; every one feels them in body and mind. The fact of our having a physical frame and an external social environment makes it certain that every one will have the feeling of inferiority in face of the outside world. Hereditary organic defects are all too frequent for complete immunity from the harsh demands of life. The environmental factors that influence a child are not the sort that make it easy for him to construct a 'correct' style of life. Pampering and imagined or actual neglect, especially pampering, all too often mislead the child into setting himself in opposition to social feeling. Moreover, the child finds his law of movement for the most part without any proper guidance. He employs the deceptive rule of trial and error with a free, personal choice that is limited only by the bounds of human possibility; but at the same time he is always struggling towards a goal of superiority which has countless variants. The child's creative energy 'uses' all impressions and sensations in building up his lasting attitude to life, in developing his individual law of movement. This fact, brought into prominence by Individual Psychology, was afterwards denoted 'attitude' or 'configuration' (*Gestalt*) without doing justice to the individual as a whole and to his close connection with the three great problems of life and without acknowledging what Individual Psychology had accomplished in this direction. Is 'neurosis' then a conflict along with all its physical and psychical consequences—the conflict of a 'difficult' child, of a suicide, of a criminal, of an arch-reactionary, of a senseless, ultra-radical fanatic, of a slack person who lives from hand to mouth, of a debauchee whose comfort has been disturbed by the distress around him? All these persons in their erroneous law of movement, to which they cling, come into conflict with 'truth' as emphasized by Individual Psychology, with 'right' seen *sub specia aeternitatis*, with the inexorable demands of an ideal community. They certainly feel the thousandfold consequences of this impact in its innumerable variants, both physical and psychical. But is this neurosis? If there were no inexorable demands of an ideal community, if every one were able in life to satisfy his mistaken law of movement—or to use a more fantastic mode of expression

—if he could satisfy his instincts, his conditioned reflexes, then there would be no conflict. No one could make such an absurd demand. It is only put forward timidly when the connection between the individual and the community is overlooked, or when an attempt has been made to separate them. Every one submits more or less willingly to the iron law of the ideal community. Only a child who has been utterly spoiled will expect and demand: 'res mihi subigere conor,' in Horace's words of reproof. A free translation of this phrase would be: 'to make use of the contributions of the community for my own ends without adding anything myself.' 'Why should I love my neighbour?' is a question that is implied in the bond that links human beings inseparably to one another in the ideal of society that leads us on inexorably.[1] He alone who has in himself and in his law of movement a sufficient tincture of this social aim and for whom it is as natural as breathing will be able to meet his approaching conflicts in the spirit of community.

The neurotic person, like every one else, has his conflicts. It is his attempt at solving them that distinguishes him clearly from all other people. Partial neuroses and mixed formations are constantly to be found in the thousandfold variants of this attempt. The neurotic, from childhood onwards, is trained in his law of movement to retreat from tasks that might, as he fears, through his failing in them injure his self-esteem and

[1] cf. also 'Der Sinn des Lebens', *Zeitschrift für Individualpsycholgie*, (1931), page 161 sqq.

interfere with his struggle for personal superiority, his struggle to be first—a struggle that is completely dissociated from social feeling. His life-motto, 'all or nothing' (as a rule very slightly modified), the excessive sensitiveness of a person continually threatened with defeats—the impatience, the intensified affects of one who lives as though he were in a hostile country, his greed—all these evoke more frequent and more violent conflicts and make the retreat that has been prescribed for him by his style of life easier. This tactical retreat, trained and tested from the days of childhood, can easily take on the deceptive appearance of a 'regression' to infantile wishes. But the neurotic is not concerned with such wishes; he is thinking only of his retreat, and he is willing to pay for this with every sort of sacrifice. Here, too, there is a possibility of mistaking these sacrifices for 'forms of self-punishment'. But, again, the neurotic is not concerned with self-punishment; he is looking for the relief he is to gain from his retreat, which will protect him from the collapse of his self-esteem and pride.

Perhaps the importance for Individual Psychology of the problem of 'security' will now at last be grasped. It can only be understood when it is seen in its whole context. It is not to be regarded as of 'secondary', but of 'primary' importance. The neurotic person 'secures' himself by his retreat, and he 'secures' his retreat by intensifying the physical and psychical shock-symptoms that have resulted from the impact of a problem that has threatened him with defeat.

WHAT REALLY IS A NEUROSIS?

He prefers his suffering to the breakdown of his sense of personal worth, of whose strength only Individual Psychology has hitherto had any knowledge. This sense of great personal worth, which is often only to be clearly seen in psychosis—this superiority complex, as I have called it—is so strong that the neurotic himself has only fear and trembling when he suspects its existence. He would gladly turn his attention away from it when he ought to put it to the test of reality. It drives him forward. But, in order to secure his retreat, he has to reject everything and forget everything that would stand in the way of that retreat. He has room only for thoughts, feelings, and actions that are concerned with his retreat.

The neurotic centres his whole interest on the retreat. Every forward step is envisaged by him as a fall into the abyss, with all its terrors. For that reason he strives with all his might, with all his feelings, and with all his tried and tested means of withdrawal, to stand firmly in the rear. He magnifies his experience of shock, turning his whole attention to it, and thereby excluding the only factor that is of importance—his fear of knowing how far away he still is from his lofty, egotistic goal. He makes large use of whipped-up emotions, for the most part in the metaphorical disguise beloved of dreams, in order to persist in his own style of life against the dictates of common sense. He is thus enabled to cling fast to his securities, which are now completely established, and which keep him from being driven on towards defeat. The opinions and the judgement of other people become

a very great danger. They admit extenuating circumstances on the outbreak of the neurosis, but if these were
absent they would not recognize the insecure nimbus
of the neurotic. In a word: *the exploiting of the experiences
of shock for the protection of the threatened nimbus*—that is
neurosis. Or still more briefly: the attitude of the neurotic person resolves itself into a 'yes-but'. In the 'yes'
there is the recognition of social feeling; in the 'but' the
retreat and the means of securing it. An injury is done
to religion when its shortcomings are made responsible
for neurosis. An injury is done to any political
party when adherence to it is cried up as a cure for
neurosis.

When our patient had left the university he tried to
find employment in a lawyer's office. He remained there
only a few weeks because his sphere of activity did not
seem worthy of him. After having made several changes
for this and for other reasons, he determined to devote
himself rather to theoretical studies. He was invited to
give lectures on legal questions, but he declined, 'because
he could not speak to large audiences'. At that time—
he was then thirty-two years old—his symptoms reap-
peared. A friend who wished to help him offered to give
a joint lecture with him. Our patient made it a condition that he should speak first. He mounted the platform
trembling and confused, and was afraid he would lose
consciousness. He saw nothing but black specks before
his eyes. Shortly after the lecture the troubles in the
region of the stomach recurred, and he imagined he
would die if he had ever to address a crowd of people

again. In the period immediately following this all he attempted was the teaching of children.

A doctor whom he consulted told him he would need to have sexual intercourse if he was to get well. The senselessness of such advice might have been foreseen. The patient, who was already retreating, reacted to the advice with the dread of syphilis, with moral scruples, and with the fear of being deceived and being saddled with the paternity of an illegitimate child. His parents advised him to marry. Their advice was apparently followed, as they found a girl for him, whom he married. His wife, when she became pregnant, left his house and returned to her parents, since, as she said, she could no longer stand his perpetual, condescending criticism.

We see now how arrogant our patient could be, given the slightest opportunity—but also how he immediately betook himself to retreat when the element of uncertainty entered into any question. He did not trouble himself about his wife and child. His sole interest lay in not appearing to be inferior, and this preoccupation was stronger than his striving for the success he desired so much. He came to grief when he drew near the front line in life, fell into a permanent state of the most intense anxiety, and strengthened his impulse to retreat by conjuring up bogies, since they made the retreat easier for him.

Are stronger proofs required? We shall give them in two different ways. In the first place we intend to work back to the period of his earliest childhood in order to

175

establish the fact that he was misled into adopting the style of life we have found him to possess. In the second place we mean to produce from his life further contributory facts that point in the same direction. In every case I should regard it as the strongest evidence of the correctness of our diagnosis if it turned out that the other contributions to our knowledge of a person's characteristics were in perfect harmony with what had been already discovered. If they should not be, then the view of the examiner has to be altered accordingly.

According to the patient his mother was of a gentle disposition. He was very much attached to her, and she thoroughly spoiled him. Moreover, she always expected very great things from him. His father was less inclined to pamper him, but he invariably yielded to the patient's wishes when he began to cry. His favourite among the other members of his family was a younger brother, who idolized him, did all he wanted him to do, ran after him like a dog, and put himself always under his guidance. The patient was the hope of the family and he always had his own way with the rest of his brother and sisters. So he was placed in an uncommonly easy and comfortable situation that unfitted him for contact with the outside world.

This was at once seen when he had to go to school for the first time. He was the youngest in his class, and he made this the excuse for showing his dislike of an inferior position by changing his school twice. But after that he showed an extraordinary eagerness to outstrip all the other pupils. When he failed to do this he beat

176

a retreat and stayed away from school on account of headaches and pains in the stomach, or he would often arrive too late. If during this period he was not among the best scholars both he and his parents attributed this to his frequent absences, while at the same time our patient strongly emphasized the fact that he knew more and had read more than all the other pupils.

His parents sent him to bed on the slightest pretext and nursed him with great tenderness. He had always been a timid child and he often cried out in his sleep in order to get his mother to occupy herself with him during the night as well as by day.

It is evident that he had no clear idea himself of the significance and the connection of all these symptoms. They were all the expression and the utterance of his style of life. Nor was he aware that he lay reading in bed until the early hours in order to enjoy the privilege on the following day of getting up at a late hour and in this way absolving himself from a part of his daily tasks. He was even more shy with girls than he was with men, and this attitude lasted during his whole development into manhood. It can be easily understood that his courage failed him in every situation in life, and that he was unwilling on any account to risk the downfall of his vanity. His uncertainty about his success with women was in strong contrast to the certainty with which he allowed himself to expect his mother's devotion. He wanted to assert in his married life the mastery which he enjoyed with his mother and his brothers and, of course, he necessarily came to grief.

WHAT REALLY IS A NEUROSIS?

I have shown that a person's style of life is to be found in the earliest memories of childhood, though they are certainly often deeply buried. Our patient's earliest recollection was the following: 'A little brother of mine had died and my father sat outside the house and wept bitterly.' We remember how the patient fled home from a lecture and gave himself up for dead.

A person's attitude to friendship is a very clear sign of his capacity for life in common with his fellow men. Our patient admits that he kept his friends only for a short time and that he invariably wanted to dominate them. This could certainly be described as nothing else than the exploitation of other people's friendship. When this was pointed out to him in a kindly manner, he answered: 'I don't believe any one works for the community; every one acts for himself alone.' The following facts show how he prepared himself for his retreat. He wanted very much to write articles or a book, but when he began to write he became so agitated that he could not think. He explains that he cannot sleep unless he reads beforehand. But when he begins to read he feels such a pressure in his head that he cannot sleep. His father died a short time before, just as the patient was visiting another town. He was to have taken up a post there a little later. He refused this on the pretext that he would die if he had to enter that town. When he was offered a situation in his own town he declined it, saying that he would not be able to sleep the first night and would therefore fail on the following day. He would have to get well first.

178

WHAT REALLY IS A NEUROSIS?

We shall now give an example of how the patient's law of movement—his 'yes-but'—is to be found in his dreams as well. The technique of Individual Psychology enables us to discover the dynamics of a dream. A dream tells us nothing new—nothing we cannot find just as well in the patient's behaviour. By the use of properly understood methods and by a selection from the content of the dream one can recognize how the dreamer, guided by his law of movement, is at pains to carry out his style of life in opposition to common sense by artificially stimulating his emotions. One often finds, too, indications that the patient is creating symptoms under the pressure of the fear of a defeat. One dream of the patient's was as follows: 'I was supposed to be visiting friends who lived on the other side of a bridge. The railing of the bridge was freshly painted in bright colours. I wanted to look into the water and leaned against the railing. This gave me a jolt on the stomach which began to give me pain. I said to myself: "You shouldn't look down into the water. You might fall in." But I took the risk for all that and went up to the railing again. I looked down and then ran quickly back, considering it was better to remain in safety.'

The visit to his friends and the freshly painted railing are indications of social feeling and of the building anew of a better style of life. The patient's fear of falling down from his height—his 'yes-but'— stand out clearly enough. As we have already pointed out, the pains in the stomach due to his feeling of fear are, as the result of his physical constitution, always at hand. The dream shows us the patient's attitude of refusal towards the efforts made by the doctor up till then and the victory of his old style of life, and this is helped by an impressive image of the danger threatening him if there is any doubt about the security of his retreat.

Neurosis is the patient's automatic, unknowing exploitation of the symptoms resulting from the effects of a shock. This exploitation is more feasible for those persons who have a great dread of losing their prestige and who have been tempted, in most cases by being pampered, to take this course. A few more observations may be added regarding the physical symptoms. In dealing with this subject certain authors celebrate imaginary triumphs. The position is as follows: the organism is a unity and has had freely presented to it by evolution the gift and dowry of a struggle for equilibrium, which is preserved as far as possible under difficult conditions. This equilibrium is maintained by the susceptibility of the pulse to variation, by the depth of the breathing, the number of respirations, the liability of the blood to congeal, and the co-operation of the endocrine glands. It becomes more and more evident in this connection that, in particular, psychical agitations affect the vegetative and the endocrine systems and occasion either an increased or a modified amount of secretion. At the present time we understand best the changes in the thyroid gland due to the effects of shock.

These changes may sometimes be fatal. I have seen such patients myself. Zondek, the greatest investigator in this field, asked me for my co-operation in determining what psychical effects are involved in these changes. Moreover, there is no question but that all cases of exophthalmic goitre develop as the result of psychical shocks. There are certain people whose thyroid gland is irritated by psychical disturbances.

Advances, too, have been made in research concerning the irritation of the suprarenal gland. It is possible to speak of a sympathetic adrenalin complex. During angry emotions, especially, the secretion of the suprarenal gland is increased. The American investigator, Cannon, has proved by experiments with animals that outbursts of anger cause an increase in the amount of adrenalin. This leads to a quickening of the heart's action and to other changes. Hence it can be understood that headaches, facial pains, perhaps even epileptic attacks, can have a psychical cause. In such cases we are dealing with people who are always irritated afresh by their problems. It is clear that here the time of life has to be taken into account. When we are dealing with a nervous girl of twenty we may assume that in her case she is threatened with problems connected with her occupation, if not with love. With a man or woman of fifty it will not be difficult to conjecture that it is the problem of growing old that the person in question imagines he or she cannot solve, or is really unable to solve. We never feel the facts of life directly, but only through our conception of them; that is the standard.

The cure can only be effected by intellectual means, by the patient's growing insight into his mistake, by the development of his social feeling.

CHAPTER XI

SEXUAL PERVERSIONS

I hope that the purely schematic account of sexual perversions given here will not cause any disappointment.[1] My main reason for hoping this is that the majority of my readers will be acquainted with the fundamental conceptions of Individual Psychology, so that tentative suggestions of a problem will be received in the same manner as a detailed treatment of it. We are more concerned here in showing that there is no discord between our outlook on the world and the structure of sexual perversions. In our generation the discussion of this question is by no means a safe matter, for precisely at the present day there is an overwhelming tendency to trace sexual perversions back to inherited factors. This is a fact of such significance that the point of view cannot be ignored. According to our conception, in sexual perversions we are dealing with artificial products that have found a place in a person's education without his knowledge. Hence it is easy to see the great contrasts

1 cf. Dreikurs, *Seelische Impotenz* (Hirzel, Leipzig), and Adler, *Das Problem der Homosexualität* (Hirzel, Leipzig, 1930).

between our views and that of other investigators. It will also be realized that our difficulties are not diminished when others, for example, Kraepelin, take up a similar position.

In order to throw light on our attitude towards other investigators I will give an account of a case which, although it has nothing to do with sexual perversions, will serve as an illustration of my psychological point of view. It is the case of a woman who lives a happy married life and has two children. For six years she has been in conflict with her environment, and this is her problem: she asserts that a woman with whom she had been friendly for many years, whom she had known since childhood and admired for her capabilities, has in the last six years developed a domineering temper and is always bent on tormenting other persons. She says that she herself has been the worst sufferer from this and brings forward in support of her statement a large number of proofs, which other people denied. She maintains: 'It is possible that in some respects I have gone too far, but in the main I am right. Six years ago this friend made some unpleasant remarks about another friend in her absence, while to her face she always pretended to be very affectionate.' Hence our patient was afraid that her friend would also make similar remarks about her. In further proof she told how her friend had said: 'The dog is no doubt obedient, but it is stupid.' She followed this up with a glance at our patient, as much as to say: 'Just like you.' The patient's acquaintances were greatly annoyed at her taking the words in such a way, for they attached no importance to them and they stoutly defended the woman who had been accused.

This woman showed her most charming side to those acquaintances. In confirmation of her opinion the patient said: 'Look how she treats her dog. She tortures him and makes him do tricks that he finds frightfully difficult.' Her neighbours replied; 'That's only a dog. You can't compare it with human beings. She is kind enough to them.' My patient's children took the friend's part very vigorously and contradicted their mother. Her husband, too, denied that any other view was possible. The patient continued to find fresh evidence of her friend's domineering attitude, which was specially directed against her. I did not hesitate to tell the patient that I thought she was right. She was overjoyed. After that other proofs followed that showed the friend's domineering disposition and the impression I had received was ultimately confirmed by the husband. Then one saw definitely that the poor woman had been quite right, only she had made a wrong use of her knowledge. Instead of understanding that we all had a more or less disguised tendency to disparage other people, and that every one should be credited with the possession of some good qualities, she turned utterly against this woman, found fault with everything she did, and became furious about it. She had a thinner skin than the others, and was able to make a better guess at what went on in her friend's mind, even if she could not understand it.

What I mean to illustrate is this: it is often the most

184

disastrous thing in the world to be in the right. This sounds a surprising statement; but perhaps every one has known from his own experience that, though right was on his side, wrong has sprung from it. One has only to imagine what might have happened to this woman if she had fallen into the hands of a less sensitive consultant. He would have spoken of persecution mania and paranoid ideas and would have treated her in such a way that she would have grown worse and worse. It is difficult to abandon one's point of view when one is in the right. This is the position of all investigators who are convinced that they are right and have their views challenged. We need not be surprised that burning quarrels should break out over our views as well; let us only be on our guard against merely being in the right and against making a wrong use of this position. We shall not allow ourselves to be irritated by the fact that so many investigators challenge our views. The scientist needs an extraordinary amount of patience. At the present day the idea of heredity has a predominant place in connection with sexual perversions. The supporters of this view may be believers in heredity pure and simple who speak of a third sex or think that this third sex exists in every one at birth; or they may be those who hold that hereditary factors come to be developed and that nothing can be done to prevent this; others again may speak of inborn physical components. None of these factors, however, can induce us to abandon our conception. It is apparent that the supporters of the organic theory in their search for organic changes and organic anomalies show up very badly.

With regard to homosexuality I should like to refer to a communication which appeared last year and which deals with this problem. The question was raised in 1927, when Laqueur found that hormones of the other sex were found in all masculine urine. This fact will make a great impression on any who do not completely grasp our conception. They might easily imagine that if perversions develop they have their origin in this dual nature of sex. But Brun's researches in connection with nine homosexuals have shown that the same hormones occur in them as in persons who are normal. That is a step forwards in our direction. Homosexuality does not depend on hormones.

I will suggest a plan according to which all the tendencies in psychology may be classified. There are *possession (Besitz) psychologies* which are occupied in showing what a human being brings with him into the world and has as his possession. From this inheritance they seek to derive all that is psychical. Seen from the standpoint of common sense this is an awkward proposition. In ordinary life people are not inclined with regard to other matters, to draw conclusions from anything a person possesses, but from the *use* he makes of it. Use interests us far more than possession. If a person possesses a sword, that does not mean that he is making a proper use of it. He can throw it away, he can slash about with it, he can whet it, etc. It is the use to which he puts it that interests us. For that reason I should like to say that there are other schools of psychology that must be regarded as *use (Gebrauch) psychologies*. Individual Psychology, which in order to understand an individual puts in the forefront his attitude to the problems of life, devotes special attention to use. For every right-thinking person I need not add that use cannot go beyond a person's capacities, and is always restricted to the bounds of human possibility, about whose range we can say nothing final. It is regrettable, and is a proof of the victorious incursion of ignoramuses into the territory of psychology, that it should still be necessary to mention such a commonplace.

With regard to the use of human abilities there is this further to be said: it was certainly the boldest step that Individual Psychology took when it asserted that in a person's psychical life the law of movement was the decisive factor in determining his individuality. Although it was necessary to have movement fixed in order to see it as form, we have always looked at everything with the conviction that all is movement, and we have found that this must be so if we are to find the solution of our problems and overcome our difficulties. It cannot be objected that the pleasure-principle contradicts this; for even the striving for pleasure is an attempt to overcome a deficiency or a feeling of pain. If this theory is correct then we shall have to look at sexual perversions also in this light. Thus only will the field of movement be illumined in the way that Individual Psychology requires. I should like to emphasize the fact that, although by this means we reach formulae and basic conceptions with regard to the structure of perversions, we have a great deal more still to do in order to understand each individual case. Every single case represents something unique, something that will never occur again. When, for example, we begin to treat a case we must discard all generalizations. From the fact that our method is a psychology of use, it follows that the human being when he is separated from his normal social environment can reveal nothing of his individuality. We shall not be able to say anything about his idiosyncrasy until we subject him to a test and then observe the use he makes of his capacities. In this respect Individual Psychology has approached the much more restricted experimental psychology, only in the case of the former it is life itself that makes the experiments. The exogenous factors with which the individual has to deal are of the greatest importance for our study of his case. We have to discover what exactly is the relationship of this unique individual to the problem that confronts him. We have to study two aspects of his personality and get to know in what way he moves in the face of his external problem; we try to discover how he endeavours to master it. The individual's 'gait'—his law of movement in face of a task that is always social—is the field of observation for Individual Psychology. Here we come across countless varieties and shades of difference. Amidst this vast number of variations we can only find our way by assuming temporarily something in the nature of a type, with the firm conviction, however, that what has been assumed to be typical will always show variants which have subsequently to be established. Our understanding of the typical case only illumines the field of observation; then follows the difficult task of discovering the individual himself. For this task a sensitive touch is needed, and it can be acquired. Furthermore the weight and impact of the actual problem in each individual case must be properly understood. This can only be achieved if one has got enough social experience and a sensitive empathy for the individual's style of life, rightly conceived—that is, for the wholeness of his individuality. In this law of movement which we perceive two typical forms can be distinguished. These I have described in my last two contributions to the *Journal for Individual Psychology* as the 'acquisitive' and 'the socially useful'.[1]

In addition to the other forms of movement shown by the sexual pervert when faced by the problems of love, we find the *narrowed path of advance* strikingly exemplified. It is evident that the normal width of path is not available, but that it is extraordinarily contracted, that only a part of the problem has been solved, as, for example, in fetishism. It is also of importance to recognize the fact that all these forms of movement by their exclusion of the norm have been directed to a goal of victory over feelings of inferiority. When we contemplate the movement (the use which a person makes of his capacities) towards which his conception of life is guiding him (the meaning he foists upon life without realizing it, without having put it into words or concepts), we can guess from this viewpoint what he is try-

[1] cf. Adler, *Zeitschrift für Individualpsychologie* (Hirzel, Leipzig), vol. x.

ing to conquer, what that satisfaction is that appears to him like a victory, when he fails to devote himself completely to the solving of the problem of love, but keeps at a distance from it, or moves slowly towards it and idles away his time. Here we might instance the procedure of Fabius Maximum Cunctator, who won a battle because he delayed so long; but this only shows again that there should be no rigid adherence to rules. This goal of conquest also becomes manifest in sexual neuroses (frigidity, ejaculatio-praecox, etc.). The problem is approached, but only from a distance, in a hesitant attitude without co-operation, and this does not lead to its solution. In this form of movement we also find the tendency to exclude, and this is seen most clearly in out-and-out homosexuality. In other cases also we can see it at work, for example, in fetishism and sadism. In the latter we find a strong aggressiveness that does not lead to the solution of the problem, and we can perceive a special form of hesitancy, of exclusion, in which the violent sexual excitement leads to the oppression of the other person—a vigorous assault that gives occasion for a defective, i.e. a one-sided, solution of a problem. This applies also to masochism, though here the goal of superiority must be understood as lying in two different directions. It is clear that the masochist gives his partner orders and that he feels himself in command despite his sense of weakness. At the same time he excludes the possibility of a defeat on a path of normal width. He achieves a victory over the *anxiety tension* by means of a trick.

190

SEXUAL PERVERSIONS

When we study the characteristic attitude of the individual we discover the following facts. When any one adheres to a definite form of movement it follows as a matter of course that he excludes other forms of the solution of the problem. This exclusion is not a mere matter of chance. Just as there has been a preparation for this mode of movement, so there has been for the exclusion as well. There can be no sexual perversion without preparation. This naturally is recognized only by those who study movement. There is still another viewpoint that we must bring sharply into prominence. The normal mode of movement would be to attack a problem in order to solve it completely, but we do not find any preparation for this when we study the pervert's previous movement. When we go back to the earliest years of a person's childhood we find that at this period, under the stimulus of external influences, a prototype has been formed from inherited capacities and potentialities. But we cannot say beforehand what this child will fashion from all the influences and experiences of his organs.[1] Here the child works in a realm of freedom with his own creative power. We find probabilities existing there in great abundance. I have always taken pains to emphasize these probabilities, and at the same time to deny that they are causally determined. It is not right to assume that a child who comes into the world with weak endocrine organs will necessarily become a neurotic, but there is a definite probability that,

[1] cf. Holub, *Die Lehre von der Organminderwertigkeit* (Hirzel, Leipzig).

191

in general, certain experiences will manifest themselves in an approximately similar way if the proper educative influences have been lacking to make social contact effective. There exist here a thousand possibilities in the realm of free choice and of error. Every one will produce some faulty formation, since no one is in possession of absolute truth. It is evident that the prototype, in order to be approximately like the normal human being, must be furnished with a definite impulse toward co-operation. A person's whole development depends on how much of the sense of contact he has acquired in his third, fourth, and fifth years. Even by this time the degree of his ability to make contact with other persons is evident. When failures are examined with this end in view it is seen that all faulty forms of movement are to be explained by lack of capability for contact. More than that—the person in question, on account of his characteristic disposition, is compelled *to protest* against every other form of movement for which he has not been prepared. We have to be tolerant in our judgement of such people, because they have never learned to develop the requisite amount of social interest. Any one who understands this knows also that the problem of love is a social problem and cannot be solved by a person who brings with him little interest in his partner, or by any one who does not have the conviction that he has a part to play in the development of humanity. He will have a different law of movement from that of the person who has been suitably prepared for the solution of the problem of love. Thus we can assert with regard to all perverts that they have not become fellow workers.

We can also discover the sources of error that enable us to understand why the child has been mistakenly held fast in the defective capacity for contact. The one fact in our social existence providing the strongest motive for this defective capacity to associate with other persons is *pampering*. Spoiled children come into contact only with the person who is spoiling them, and as a result they are forced to exclude every one else. Still other influences are to be noted in connection with each particular perversion. One can put it like this: here the child as a result of this experience has formed his law of movement in such a way that he has settled the question of his relationship to the other sex in this particular manner. All perverts show their law of movement not only in relation to the problem of love, but on the occasion of every test for which they have not been prepared. For that reason we find among perverts all the character-traits of neurosis—hypersensitiveness, impatience, a tendency to outbursts of anger, covetousness, as well as the attempt to justify themselves by saying that they act as though they were under compulsion. They have a certain keen desire to possess which leads them to carry out the plan implied in their characteristic disposition, and the result is that one finds so violent a protest against any other form of movement that even dangers to other persons are not entirely excluded (rape, sadism).

I should like to show how the preparation for a given form of perversion is discovered. I will give an example which indicates that certain perversions may come into existence as the result of such training. We must not seek for the preparation in the region of the material alone, we have to understand that it can be carried on in the world of thought and of dreams. Individual Psychology lays great stress on this, because many believe, for example, that a perverse dream is a proof of innate homosexuality, while we are able from our conception of the dream-life to establish that this homosexual dream is part of the preparation, precisely as it has its part also in the development of interest in the same sex and the exclusion of interest in the other sex. I shall give an example of this training in a case where, owing to the age of the individual, there can be no question of sexual perversions. I cite two dreams in order to show that the law of movement is found in the dream-life as well. If one is equipped with a knowledge of Individual Psychology he will not be afraid to search for the whole life-pattern in every minute fragment of it. We must, however, find the whole life-pattern in the content of the dream and not merely in the dream-thoughts, though certainly these thoughts, if we understand them properly and relate them correctly to the style of life, are of extraordinary assistance to our knowledge of the individual's attitude to the problem confronting him— an attitude into which he has been inexorably forced by his style of life. I should like to point out that what we are doing here is like the work of a detective. We are not fortunate enough to be in possession of all the material facts that are indispensable. We have to exercise to the very utmost our ability to conjecture in order to construct the unity of the individual.

The first dream:

'I imagined I was in the next war. All the men, and even all the boys over ten years old had to enlist. . . .'

From the first sentence the Individual Psychologist can conclude that this is a child whose attention is centred on the dangers of life and on the ruthlessness of other persons.

'. . . Then it happened that one evening I awoke to find myself in a hospital bed. My parents were sitting beside the bed.'

His choice of an image shows that he has been pampered.

'I asked them what was the matter. They said there was a war. They did not want the war to affect me so badly so they had had an operation performed to turn me into a girl.'

From this it can be seen how anxious his parents were about him. He means: when I am in danger I cling to my parents. That is the expressive form of a spoilt child. We shall not take any step in advance if we cannot do so unconditionally. We are bound to be as sceptical as possible in our work. The problem of sex metamorphosis emerges here. Apart from scientific attempts that are still very questionable, it must be said that the possibility of transforming a boy into a girl is credited only by the layman. In this dream we find uncertainty with regard to sex-life. It shows us that the dreamer is not

195

quite certain about his sexual role. This will surprise
many when they learn that this was a youth of twelve
years. We shall be able to observe how he came to have
this idea. Life appears to him to be unacceptable on
account of its problems such as that of war; he protests
against it.

'Girls don't have to go to war. If I were to enlist my
genitals could not be shot off, since I haven't got any
like the other boys.'

In war the genitals are endangered—a not very obvious argument in favour of castration, or perhaps it
gives expression to his social feeling in an aversion to
war.

'I came home, but as by a miracle the war had
stopped.'

So the operation was unnecessary. What will he do
now?

'Perhaps it isn't necessary that I should be like a
girl. Perhaps there won't be any war.'

We see that he does not quite give up his role as a
boy. We must take note of that in connection with his
law of movement. He tries to go a little further in the
direction of masculinity.

'At home I was very unhappy and I cried a great
deal.'

Children who cry a great deal have been spoiled.

'When my parents asked me why I was crying I said
I was afraid that as I belonged to the female sex I would
have to suffer the pains of child-birth when I got older.'

So the female role, too, was of no use. We were on the

right track for the discovery of his goal when we assumed thatthe youthwanted to avoid all unpleasant situations. I have found in the case of sexual perverts that as children they had been spoiled and often kept in ignorance. They have, to say the least, a great craving for appreciation, for immediate success, and for personal superiority. In such a case it is quite likely that a child does not know whether he is a boy or a girl. What ought he to do? He sees no hope either as a boy or a girl.

'The next day I went to my club, for in real life I am a member of a Pathfinder Club.'

We can already imagine how he will behave himself there.

'I dreamed that there was one solitary girl at our club. She stood apart from the boys.'

This is an attempt to form a definite distinction between the sexes.

'The boys cried to me to come over to them. I said I was a girl and I went to this girl who was alone. It seemed very strange to me that I wasn't any longer a boy, and I wondered how I should have to behave as a girl.'

Suddenly the question arises: *How should I have to behave as a girl?*

This is the training. Only those who have noted the training in all sexual perversions and seen how it is forced away from the normal by elimination will understand that sexual perversion is an artificial product. Each person has formed it for himself; he has been directed to it by the psychical constitution he has him-

197

self created and has occasionally been misled into it by his inherited physical constitution which makes the deviation easier for him.

'As I thought this over I was disturbed by a crash. I woke up and found I had hit my head against the wall.'

The dreamer often assumes the position that corresponds to his law of movement.[1] To run one's head against a brick wall is a popular saying. His whole attitude leads us to expect this result.

'The dream made such a deep impression on me,' it is the purpose of a dream to leave an impression behind it, 'that when I went back to school I was still uncertain whether I was a boy or a girl. In the intervals I had to go to the lavatory to see if I wasn't a girl after all.'

The second dream:
'I dreamed I met the only girl in our class. It was the same girl I had dreamt about before. She wanted to go for a walk with me. I replied: I only go with boys. She said: "I'm a boy, too." As this did not seem likely to me I asked her to prove it to me. Then she showed me that she had an organ like a boy's. I asked her how that could be possible. She told me she had had an operation. It was easier for boys to be changed into girls than the other way round, because something had to be added. So she had sewn on a boy's organ made of rubber. But at that moment our talk was broken off by a loud "get up". My parents had wakened me. It was only with

[1] cf. Adler, 'Schlafstellungen' in *Praxis und Theorie der Individualpsychologie* (Bergmann, Munich, 4th edition).

trouble and difficulty I could get five minutes' grace, but as I am no wizard I could not bring the dream back again.'

An inclination to magic is to be found in a certain type of spoilt children. Magic seems to them to be of primary importance. They want to have everything without any exertion or trouble and they have plenty of time for telepathy.

We shall now hear how this youth attempts to explain this dream to himself.

'I have read in stories about the war of genitals flying through the air. I have heard that when any one loses his genitals he dies.'

One can see the importance this youth attaches to the genitals.

'I read on the front page of a newspaper: "Two housemaids changed into soldiers in two hours." '

This may possibly have been a case of malformation of the sexual organs that had been misunderstood.

In conclusion I should like to say something that puts all the discussions relevant to this topic on a simpler basis. There are genuine hermaphrodites with whom it is really difficult to say whether one is dealing with girls or boys. They can decide for themselves what use they make of their hermaphroditism. Among the pseudo-hermaphrodites there are to be found malformations that have a deceptive similarity to the organ of the other sex. The fact is that every human being carries in him traces of the other sex, just as there are also hormones of the other sex in the urine. This gives occasion for a surmise that seems rather bold: viz. that there is a twin hidden in every one of us. Twinship is marked by the most varied of forms, and the possibility of the simultaneous existence of two sexual forms in human beings will be decided when the problem of twinship is solved. We know that every human being is born from male and female material. It is quite possible that in the investigation of the question of twinship we may come across problems which will throw more light on the hermaphroditism present in every person.

A sentence or two may be added with reference to the treatment. One hears constantly that a perversion is incurable. The cure of perverts is not impossible but it is difficult. The difficulty of the cure is due to the fact that they are persons who during their whole life have been trained for perversion because they have a restricted law of movement which prescribes this course for them. They have to move in this direction because from their earliest youth they have not found the contact that would enable them to make the proper use of their body and mind. The proper use of these can be ensured only if there has been beforehand a developed social feeling. It is a knowledge of this fact that makes the cure *even of the majority of perverts* seem quite probable.

In the following explanation, which seems to me quite valid, I will attempt to show that the sexual function, like all other functions, begins without social interest. Eating, excreting, looking, hearing, talking, are in the beginning only controlled by the needs of the child's body. The ordinary educative and cultural influences assist the child's creative powers to bring about an accord between his functions and the demands of social life. The degree of social interest gained by the child will decide the extent to which this accord will be attained, and whether the child is to be a help or a burden. The same social interest is valuable in regard to the sexual function, which in the beginning of life is a function for *one* person and is clearly expressed in masturbation. The slow development of this function and a lack of conditions favourable to its growth into a social function—i.e. when it is a task for two persons of different sexes—obstruct its right evolutionary development for love and procreation and for the preservation of mankind. The degree of social interest determines the issue. All forms of perversions and deficiencies are varieties of masturbation, representing the first phase of the sexual function. Proof of this can be found in the style of life of all perverts and in the manner in which they relate themselves to outside problems.

CHAPTER XII

EARLIEST RECOLLECTIONS OF
CHILDHOOD

However little we know of the unity of the ego we can never get away from it. It is possible to analyse the homogeneous psychic life in accordance with various more or less valueless points of view; two or three spatial conceptions that are meant to explain the indivisible ego may be compared or contrasted with one another. The attempt may be made to unfold this unity from the conscious, from the unconscious, from the sexual, or from the external world; but in the end there can be no evading the necessity of restoring it again to its all-embracing activity, like setting a rider once more on his steed. Nevertheless the progress made on the path that Individual Psychology has blazed can no longer be misunderstood. The ego, in the view of modern psychology, has established its worth, and whether or not it is believed to have been turned out of its quarters in the unconscious or in the 'Id', in the end the 'Id' behaves itself with good or bad manners, just like the ego. Even the so-called conscious, or the ego, is chock-full of the unconscious, or, as I have called it, the not-understood, and it always shows varying degrees of social feeling. These facts have been more and more realized and incorporated in an artificial system by psycho-analysis, which has made of Individual Psychology 'a prisoner that will never set it free'.

It can be easily understood that at a very early stage of my endeavours to throw light on the impregnable unity of the psychic life I had to reckon with the function and the structure of memory. I was able to confirm the statements of earlier writers that memory is by no means to be regarded as the gathering-place of impressions and sensations; that impressions are not retained as 'mneme', but that in the function of memory we are dealing with a partial expression of the power of the homogenous psychical life—of the ego. The ego, like perception, has the task of fitting impressions into the completed style of life and using them in accordance with it. To use a cannibalistic simile, one might say that the task of memory is to devour and digest impressions. I do not need to point out to my readers that they should not immediately conclude from this simile that memory has a sadistic tendency. The digestive process, however, is the function of the style of life. Anything that does not suit its palate is discarded, forgotten, or kept as a warning example. The decision rests with the style of life. If it is taken up with warnings, it uses the indigestible impressions for that purpose. In this connection one is reminded of the character-trait of caution. A good deal is half-digested; sometimes only a quarter or a thousandth part is accepted. But the process can also take the line of digesting only those feelings and states of mind that accompany the impressions. With these there are occasionally mingled memories of words or ideas or fragments of them. Suppose I forget the name of a person otherwise well known to me. He need not necessarily always be a person whom I dislike, nor need he remind me of anything disagreeable; so far, too, as his name and his personality are concerned, these may lie, either for the present or permanently, outside the interest that has been thrust upon them by my style of life; still I often know everything connected with him that seems to be of importance. He stands before me. I can place him and say a great deal about him. Precisely because I cannot remember his name he stands out fully and clearly in my conscious field of vision. That means that my memory can let portions of the whole impression or the whole of the impression itself disappear, for one of the purposes already described or for some other purpose. This is an artistic ability that corresponds to an individual's style of life. Therefore the impression as a whole includes much more than the experience that has been clothed in words. The individual apperception hands over to the memory the observed facts that are in accordance with the individual's characteristic disposition. He is led by his idiosyncrasy to take over the impression that has been formed in this way and he equips it with feelings and with a state of mind. Both the feelings and the state of mind in their turn obey the individual's law of movement. There remains over from this process of digestion what we mean to call recollection, whether that is expressed in words or feelings or in an attitude to the external world. This process more or less includes what we understand by the function of memory. An ideal, objective reproduction of impressions independent of the individual's idiosyncrasy therefore does not exist. We must accordingly expect to reckon on finding just as many forms of memory as there are forms of the style of life.

I give one of the commonest examples of a definite life-pattern and the memory connected with it which should illustrate this fact.

A man complained very bitterly that his wife forgot 'everything'. A doctor would at once think of some organic trouble in the brain. Since that was out of the question in this case, I proceeded to make an exhaustive inquiry into the patient's style of life, provisionally leaving the symptom out of account—a necessity that many psychotherapeutists do not recognize. She proved to be a quiet, amiable, intelligent person who had managed to get married to a domineering man in the face of difficulties caused by his parents. During the course of her married life her husband made her feel her pecuniary dependence on him as well as the fact of her humble origin. For the most part she bore his corrections and reproofs in silence. Occasionally the question of a separation had been raised by both of them. But the possibility of uninterrupted mastery over the woman kept the husband again and again from taking that extreme step.

She was the only child of kindly, affectionate parents

205

who never found anything to blame in their daughter. From her childhood she preferred to be without the company of other children when she was playing or was busy with anything. Her parents saw nothing wrong in that, particularly as she behaved herself irreproachably when she happened to be in company with other girls. But in her married life as well she was careful not to have her time for being alone, her hours for reading, her leisure, as she called it, too much broken into either by her husband or by social demands. Her husband, on the other hand, would have preferred to have more opportunities of showing how superior he was to her. Moreover, she was extraordinarily zealous in the performance of her housewifely duties. The only exception was that she failed with amazing frequency to carry out her husband's instructions.

It appeared from the recollections of her childhood that she was always extremely happy when she could perform her duties by herself.

The experienced student of Individual Psychology will see at the first glance that the patient's life-pattern was very well suited for actions she was able to carry out by herself, but not for joint tasks like love and marriage which need two persons for their proper achievement. Her husband, owing to his own idiosyncrasies, was unable to impart this power to her. Her goal of perfection lay in the direction of solitary work. When this was concerned she was blameless. And any one who only kept this side of her nature in view would have been unable to discover any fault in her. But she had not been prepared for love and marriage. She could not pull in double harness. We are able also to conjecture—to mention only one detail—that the form of her sex-life was—frigidity. And now we can proceed to consider the symptom which we rightly left provisionally out of account at first. As a matter of fact we already understand it. Her forgetfulness was the mildly aggressive form of her protest against being compelled to take part in work for which she had not been prepared, and, moreover, it lay outside her goal of perfection.

It is not every one who can recognize and understand an individual's complicated artistry from such a brief description. But the theory that Freud and his disciples —who have all to be psycho-analysed—have tried to draw from Individual Psychology is more than doubtful; it is self-condemned, since it implies that, according to our account, a patient 'only' wants to attract attention and get other people to take a greater interest in him.

Incidentally, the question is frequently raised as to whether a case is to be considered easy or difficult. According to our view this depends entirely on the degree of the patient's social feeling. In the case we are considering it is easy to understand that this woman's mistake—her imperfect preparation for life and work in common—was easier to remedy, since she had neglected the most important keystone only from forgetfulness, so to speak. She was convinced of this, and, through co-operation with the doctor in friendly talks, while her husband was being instructed by the doctor at the same time, she was delivered from her charmed circle (Künkel playfully styles it the devil's circle; Freud, the magic circle). Her forgetfulness also disappeared, since it was deprived of its motive.

We are now ready to understand that every recollection, in so far as an experience affects the individual at all and is not rejected forthwith, represents the result of the elaboration of an impression by means of the style of life, i.e. by the ego. This holds good not merely for those recollections that have been firmly retained, but also for those that are imperfect and difficult to recall, and even for those that are not expressed in words but exist only as an emotional tone or as a state of mind. We are thus able to establish a relatively important position. This implies that the observer must gain a knowledge of every form of psychical movement with its direction towards a goal of perfection by clearly establishing what is due to intellect, to emotion, and to attitude in the range of memory. As we know already, the ego expresses itself not only in speech but also in its emotions and in its attitude, and the science of the unity of the ego owes to Individual Psychology the discovery of organ-dialect. We maintain our contact with the external world by every fibre of our body and mind. What interests us in a case is the manner, especially the imperfect manner, in which this contact is maintained. Following this path I found it my fascinating and valuable task to discover and utilize the individual's recollections, in whatever way they appeared, as a significant part of his style of life. I was, above all, interested in those recollections that were regarded as the earliest. The reason was that they throw light on events, real or imagined, correctly reported or altered, that lie nearer to the creative construction of the style of life in the first years of childhood, and that also to a large extent dis-close the elaboration of these events by the style of life. Here we are not so much concerned with the actual content of the memory, for this is to be regarded simply as content for every person. We have rather to estimate its probable emotional tone, with the frame of mind re-sulting from it, and the elaboration and choice of the material with which it has been framed—this latter because it will assist us in discovering the principal interest of the individual; and that is an essential ingre-dient in his style of life. At this point the main question of Individual Psychology gives us considerable assis-tance: What is this individual's aim? What is his conception of himself and of life? We undoubtedly receive guidance from the unyielding conceptions of Individual Psychology regarding the goal of perfection, the feeling of inferiority (the knowledge of this, though not the understanding of it, as Freud recognizes, has spread over the whole world); and also from its doctrine of the inferiority and superiority complexes. But all these closely knit conceptions only serve to throw light on the field of vision in which we have to discover the par-ticular law of movement of the person with whom we are dealing.

As we set about this task we find ourselves confronted by the question that makes us doubt whether we may not easily be mistaken in our interpretation of recollections and of their connection with the style of life, since individual forms of expression may have several inter-pretations. Certainly any one who practises Individual Psychology with proper artistry will never be mistaken with regard to the special nuances. But even he will endeavour to eliminate every kind of error. And it is quite possible to do this. If he has found an individual's real law of movement in his recollections, then he must find that same law of movement in all the other forms of expression. So far as concerns the treatment of failures of all kinds he will have to produce so many proofs of these that the patient also will be convinced by the weight of the evidence. The doctor himself will be con-vinced, sometimes sooner, sometimes later, according to his individual bent. But there is no other standard by which to estimate a person's failures, his symptoms, and his mistaken mode of living than a sufficient measure of right social feeling.

Provided we use the utmost care and, possess the requisite experience we are now in a position to dis-cover, for the most part from the earliest recollections, the mistaken direction given to the style of life, and the lack, or the presence, of social feeling. Here we are guided especially by our knowledge of the lack of social feeling and by our knowledge of its causes and conse-quences. A great deal comes to light when a situation is described with the frequent use of the words 'we' and 'I'. Much, too, can be learned from the way in which the mother is mentioned. Recollections of dangers and acci-dents, as well as of corrections and penalties, disclose an exaggerated tendency to fix attention especially on the hostile element in life. The remembrance of the birth of a brother or sister reveals the situation of dethronement. The memory of the first appearance in the kindergarten or the school shows the great impression produced by new situations. The recollections of sickness or of a death is often linked with a fear of these dangers, and occasionally with the attempt to become better equipped to meet them by becoming a doctor or a nurse or by some such means. Memories of visits to the country with the mother, as well as the mention of certain persons like the mother, the father, or the grandparents in a kindly spirit, often show not only a preference for people who have evidently pampered the child, but also the exclusion of other persons. Recollections of misdeeds, thefts, and sexual misdemeanours indicate that a great effort is being made to exclude them hereafter from experience. Occasionally other trends are discovered—visual, aural, or kinaesthetic. These are very helpful in leading to the discovery of failures at school, the wrong choice of a profession, and they can also give an opportunity of suggesting a calling that will fit in better with the individual's preparation for life.

One or two examples may help to show the connection between the earliest recollections and the permanent life-pattern.

A man about thirty-two years old, the eldest, spoilt son of a widow, proves unfitted for any profession because as soon as he begins to work he is seized with severe attacks of anxiety, though these improve immediately he returns home again. He is a good-natured man, but he finds it difficult to mix with other persons. At school he became very excited before any examination, and often stayed away from school on the ground that he was tired and exhausted. His mother looked after him most affectionately. As he was properly prepared only for this maternal solicitude, it was easy to conjecture his goal of superiority, his effort to evade as far as possible all the problems of life, and thereby avoid every mistake. So long as he was with his mother there was no danger. His clinging to his mother gave him an infantile stamp, although physically there was nothing infantile to be noted about him. This method of retreating to his mother, well tested since he was a child, found notable support when the first girl to whom he took a liking rejected him. The shock he experienced as the result of this 'exogenous' event confirmed him in his desire to retreat, so that he was never at ease unless he was with his mother. His earliest recollection from childhood was the following: 'When I was about four years old I sat at the window and watched some workmen building a house on the opposite side of the street, while my mother knitted stockings.'

It may be objected that this is rather insignificant. But that is by no means the case. His *choice of the earliest memory*—whether it was really the earliest or not does not matter—shows us that some interest or other must have attracted him to it. The active work of his memory, guided by his style of life, selects an event which gives a strong indication of his individual tendency. The pampered child is revealed by the fact that the memory recalls a situation that includes the solicitous mother. But a still more important fact is disclosed. *He looks on while other people work.* His preparation for life is that of an onlooker. He is scarcely anything more than that. If he ventures beyond that he feels that he is on the brink of a precipice and beats a retreat under the effect of the shock—fear of the discovery—of his worthlessness. If he is left at home with his mother, if he is allowed to look on while others work, then there does not seem to be anything wrong with him. He aims in his line of movement at the domination of his mother as his only goal of superiority. Unfortunately there are few prospects in life for a mere onlooker. Nevertheless, after a patient like that has been cured, one will be on the lookout for some employment in which he can put to some use the better preparation of his power of seeing and observing. Since we understand his case better than the patient, we must intervene actively and let him understand that while he can get on in any calling, if he wants to make the best use of his preparation he should seek some work in which *observation is chiefly needed.* He took up successfully a business dealing with articles of vertu.

Using distorted nomenclature Freud, without realizing the fact, *invariably describes the failings of pampered children.* The spoilt child wants to have everything, and only performs with difficulty the normal functions that evolution has established. He desires his mother in his 'Oedipus complex'. (Although this is an exaggerated way of describing the condition, yet in rare cases it is intelligible, because the spoilt child rejects every other person.) In later years he meets with every kind of difficulty—not on account of the repression of the Oedipus complex, but on account of the shock he receives when confronted by other situations—and gets into such a frenzied state that he even harbours murderous designs against other persons who oppose his wishes. As can be clearly seen these artificial products of an imperfect, pampering education can only be utilized for gaining a knowledge of the psychical life, if the consequences of pampering are recognized and taken into account. Sex-life, however, is a task for two persons, which can only be rightly performed if there is a sufficient amount of social feeling present, and this is lacking in the case of spoilt children. In a crass generalization Freud is compelled to attribute to innate sadistic instincts the wishes, fantasies and symptoms that have been artificially nurtured, as well as the resistance to them offered by what remains of social feeling. These 'sadistic instincts', as we see, are the consequences of pampering and are artificially bred in the child at some later date. Hence it is easy to understand that the first act of a new-born child —drinking from the mother's breast—is co-operation, and is as pleasant for the mother as for the child. It is not cannibalism or a proof of inherited sadistic instincts, as Freud, bolstering up his preconceived theory, imagines. The great variety in the forms of human life disappears in the obscurity of the Freudian view.

Another example will show the usefulness of our

knowledge of the earliest recollections of childhood. A girl of eighteen lived in perpetual bickering with her parents. They wanted her to go on with her studies, as she had done very well at school. But she refused, because, as it turned out, she was afraid of failure, since she was not first in the school examination. Her earliest childhood's recollection was as follows. When she was four years old she had seen at a children's party another girl playing with a huge ball. Being a very pampered child, nothing would satisfy her but that she must have a ball like it. Her father searched the whole town to get one, but he was not successful. The girl was given a smaller ball, but she refused it with screams and tears. It was only after her father had explained how all his trouble had been in vain that she became quiet and accepted the smaller ball. From this recollection I was able to conclude that this girl could be influenced by friendly explanations; she could be convinced about her self-seeking ambition, and I was successful in curing her.

The following case shows how obscure the ways of fate can often be. A man of forty-two became impotent after many years of marriage with a woman who was ten years older than he. For two years he had scarcely spoken to his wife or to his two children. Although in former years he had been moderately successful in his business, since then he had neglected it and had brought his family into a lamentable condition. He was his mother's favourite son and greatly spoiled. When he was three years old a sister had been born. Shortly after that

EARLIEST RECOLLECTIONS OF CHILDHOOD

—the arrival of the sister was his earliest recollection— he began to wet the bed. And, as we often find among spoilt children, he had terrifying dreams when he was a child. There can be no question that the bed-wetting and the anxiety sprang from attempts to undo his dethronement; and in this connection we should not overlook the fact that the bed-wetting was also the expression of an accusation, perhaps more than that, of an act of revenge against his mother. At school he was a superlatively good child. He remembered the only occasion on which he had been involved in a fight, with another boy who had insulted him. The teacher said he was amazed that such a good boy could allow himself to be carried away as he had done.

We can understand that he had been trained to expect exclusive attention, and that his goal of superiority lay in his being preferred to other boys. If this did not happen he adopted measures that were partly accusing and partly revengeful, although the motive of his actions was not realized either by himself or by other persons. A great deal of his egotistically tinctured goal of perfection consisted in his not wanting to be thought a bad boy. As he said himself, he had married a girl who was older than himself because she treated him like a mother. Since she was now more than fifty years old and taken up more than ever with the care of the children, he broke off all intercourse with them in an apparently unaggressive manner. His impotence as organ dialect was connected with this rupture. One can now well understand why in the early years of his childhood, when his pampering was stopped on the birth of his sister, he constantly practised the less obvious, but none the less effective, accusation of bed-wetting.

A man of thirty, the older of two children, had to undergo a fairly long term of imprisonment for repeated thefts. His earliest recollections came from his third year—the period after the birth of his younger brother. They ran: 'My mother always preferred my brother to me. I ran away from home even when I was a little child. Occasionally, when driven by hunger, I stole some small things both in the house and outside. My mother punished me terribly. But I always ran away again. I was at school until I was fourteen, but I was only a mediocre scholar; I did not want to learn any more and I roamed about the streets alone. I was sick of home. I had no friends and I never found a girl who cared for me, although I always longed for one. I wanted to go to dancing-halls and make acquaintances there, but I hadn't any money. Then I stole a motor-car and sold it very cheaply. After this I began to steal on a bigger scale, till finally I was put in prison. Perhaps I might have chosen another mode of life if I had not been disgusted with my home, where I got nothing but abuse. My thefts, however, were encouraged by a receiver of stolen goods into whose hands I fell, and who incited me to steal.'

I have already drawn attention to the fact that in the majority of cases one finds that law-breakers have been pampered or have had a craving for pampering when they were children. Just as important, too, is the fact that one can perceive in their childhood a greater activity,which,however, is not to be mistaken for courage. The mother was capable of spoiling a child, as is shown by the way in which she dealt with the younger son. We can conclude from the embittered attitude of this man after the birth of his younger brother that he too had been spoiled. His vicissitudes in later life had their origin in his embittered complaint against his mother and in that activity for which, in the absence of a sufficient degree of social feeling—no friends, no calling, no love—he found no other outlet than in crime. To be able to come before the public, as certain psychiatrists have recently done, with the theory that crime is self-punishment combined with the wish to go to prison, really betrays a want of the sense of intellectual shame, especially when it is bound up with an open contempt for common sense and with insulting attacks on our well-founded experiences. I leave it to the reader to decide whether or not such views originate in the spirit of pampered children and have their reaction on the minds of other pampered children among the members of the public.

CHAPTER XIII

SOCIALLY OBSTRUCTIVE SITUATIONS IN CHILDHOOD AND THEIR REMOVAL

In our search for situations that predispose and allure the child to take the wrong path, we come across again and again those difficult problems which I have already described as being the most important. They tend to make the development of social feeling difficult, and therefore in very many cases they also prove to be an obstacle to it. Such problems are pampering, congenital organic inferiorities, and neglect. The effects of these factors vary not merely in their extent and their degree, nor do they differ only in their duration, reckoning from the beginning to the end of their activity, but above all in the almost incalculable agitation and sense of responsibility they arouse in the child. The child's attitude to these factors depends not only on his use of trial and error, but much more, as can be proved, on his energy of growth and his creative power. This creative power is part of the life-process, and its unfolding in our civilization, which both represses and encourages the child, is also an almost incalculable factor, whose strength can only be judged from its consequences. If we wish to proceed any further by way of conjecture we must keep before our view an immense number of facts—family peculiarities, light, air, the season of the year, noise, contact with other persons who are more or less suitable, climate, nature of the soil, nutriment, the endocrine system, the muscular build, the tempo of organic development, the embryonal stage, and much else, such as the help and nursing given by the persons who have care of the child. In this perplexing array we shall be likely to assume that these factors are sometimes helpful and at other times injurious. We shall be satisfied with keeping in view with great caution statistical probabilities in each case, without denying the possibility of divergent results. There is much less chance of our being wrong if we adopt the method of observing results in which any variation is likely to occur. The child's creative power will then come to light, and we shall have ample opportunity of estimating it in the greater or less activity displayed by body and mind.

But we must not overlook the fact that the child's inclination to co-operation is challenged from the very first day. The immense importance of the mother in this respect can be clearly recognized. She stands on the threshold of the development of social feeling. The biological heritage of human social feeling is entrusted to her charge. She can strengthen or hinder contact by the help she gives the child in little things, in bathing him, in providing all that a helpless infant is in need of. Her relations with the child, her knowledge, and her aptitude are decisive factors. We are not to forget that in this regard, also human evolution in its highest attainments can effect an adjustment, and that the child itself can overcome any hindrances that may be present, compelling contact by screaming and obstinacy. For in the mother as well the biological inheritance of maternal love—an invincible portion of social feeling—lives and works. It can be obstructed by adverse conditions, excessive worries, disappointments, illness, and suffering, by a notable want of social feeling and its consequences; but the evolutionary inheritance of maternal love is usually so strong in animals and in human beings that it easily overcomes the instincts of hunger and of sex. It may be readily accepted that contact with the mother is of the highest importance for the development of human social feeling. If we renounced the use of this omnipotent lever of human development we should be extremely embarrassed to find a substitute for it that was half as effective, quite apart from the fact that the maternal sense of contact, as an evolutionary possession which cannot be lost, would relentlessly oppose its being destroyed. *We probably owe to the maternal sense of contact the largest part of human social feeling, and along with it the essential continuance of human civilization.* Certainly maternal love at the present day is often insufficient for the needs of the community. In a distant future *the use of this possession* will be far more in accordance with the social ideal. For the bond between mother and child is frequently too weak, and, still more frequently, too strong. In the former case the child may get an impression of the hostility of life from the beginning, and, as a result of similar experiences, he may make this *meaning* the plumb-line of his life.

As I have found often enough, in these cases even a better contact with the father (not with the grandparents) is sufficient to compensate for this defect. It may be asserted that as a general rule the better contact of a child with the father shows that that there has been a failure on the part of the mother, and it almost always signifies a second phase in the life of a child who, rightly or wrongly, has been disappointed in the mother. The closer contact that girls frequently have with their father and boys with their mother cannot be attributed to sexuality. This fact must be tested in reference to the statement that has just been made. Here two points are to be noted. Fathers often show a tender feeling towards their daughters, just as they are accustomed to do towards all girls and women; and both girls and boys, getting themselves ready as they do for their future life in all their games,[1] make this same playful preparation also in their attitude to the parent of the opposite sex. I have found that the sexual instinct also occasionally comes into play, though certainly not in the exaggerated fashion that Freud depicts, in the case of very spoilt children, who wish to restrict their whole development to the family circle, or, still more closely, to an exclusive attachment to a single person who pampers them. The mother's bounden duty, from the viewpoint of historical development and of society, is to make the child as early

[1] cf. Groos, *Spiele der Kinder,*

as possible a partner, a fellow being who willingly gives help and willingly allows himself to be helped when his powers are unequal to his task. Volumes could be written about the 'well-tuned' child. Here we must be content to point out that the child ought to feel himself a member with equal rights in the home, taking a growing interest in his father, his brothers and his sisters, and soon also in all other persons. Thus at an early stage he will cease to be a burden and become a partner. He will soon feel himself at home and develop that courage and confidence that spring from his contact with his environment. Any troubles he may cause, whether intentionally or not, by functional mistakes like bed-wetting, retention of faeces, difficulties in eating not caused by illness, will become problems which he himself as well as those around him will be able to solve, apart from the fact that these disorders will not make their appearance if his inclination to co-operate is strong enough. The same holds good for thumb-sucking, biting the nails, thrusting the fingers into the nose, and taking large bites of food. All these traits appear only when the child refuses to play his part and does not accept his cultural training. They are seen almost exclusively among spoilt children, and are meant to force those around them to be more active and make greater efforts on their behalf. They are also invariably combined with open or veiled obstinacy, and they are clear signs of imperfect social feeling. It is long since I drew attention to these facts. If Freud to-day tries to mitigate the fundamental conception of his doctrine—universal sexuality—this correction is due in a large measure to the experiences of Individual Psychology. The much more recent view of Charlotte Bühler with regard to a 'normal' stage of defiance has certainly to be brought into line with our experiences. It follows from the structure we have just described that the faults of childhood are bound up with character traits like obstinacy, jealousy, self-love, want of social feeling, egotistic ambition, desire for revenge, etc., and these traits are seen sometimes more, sometimes less distinctly. This also corroborates our conception of character as a guiding-line for the goal of superiority. It is a reflection of the style of life—a social attitude that is not innate, but is brought to completion simultaneously with the law of movement which the child has formed. The characteristics of spoilt children, who are unable to deny themselves any wish or enjoyment, are shown in their clinging to the probably trifling pleasures of retention of faeces, thumb-sucking, childish play with the genitals, etc., which possibly are sometimes first started for the purpose of getting rid of certain tickling sensations.

The personality of the father forms another dangerous corner in the development of social feeling. The mother should not deprive him of the opportunity of creating as permanent a relationship with the child as possible. He may easily fail to do this when there is pampering, when there is imperfect social feeling, or when the child dislikes him. He must not be singled out as the person who threatens and punishes, and he must give the child enough of his time and affection to ensure that he is not driven into the background. I might instance other acts on the father's part that are particularly harmful—his trying to supplant the mother by excessive affection, introducing a harsh régime to correct the mother's pampering, thus driving the child closer to the mother, or attempting to force his authority and his principles on the child. By this last he may induce submission, but never co-operation and social feeling. In our age of haste the mealtimes provide a special opportunity for the cultivation of communal life. A pleasant atmosphere at table is indispensable. Lectures on table-manners should be given as seldom as possible. There will be better results if this rule is observed. Fault-finding, bursts of anger, and peevishness should be avoided at the table, nor should there be any indulgence in reading or in brooding. This, too, is not the time to take children to task for failures at school or for other misdemeanours. Further, an attempt should be made to have meals in common; this seems to me to apply especially to breakfast. It is important that children should have complete freedom to speak and to ask questions. Laughing at children, mocking them, or holding other children up to them as examples of good behaviour will injure the sense of contact and may induce reserve, shyness, or some other acute feeling of inferiority. Children should not be reminded of their littleness or of their lack of knowledge and ability. They should have a clear path for a training in courage. Let them be given free scope when they show an interest in anything and do not take everything out of their hands; always tell them that it is only the beginning that is difficult, and in regard to dangers do not show excessive anxiety but take proper precaution and provide sufficient protection. Nervousness on the part of the parents, domestic quarrels, disagreements with regard to education can easily hinder the development of social feeling. A too peremptory dismissal of children from the company of grown-ups should if possible be avoided. Praise or blame should be given to success or failure in the training and not to the personality of the child.

Illness can also become a perilous obstacle to the development of social feeling. Like other difficulties it is more dangerous when it occurs in the first five years of the child's life. We have already referred to the importance of innate organic inferiorities and have shown that statistically they have proved to be evils that lead in a wrong direction and become hindrances to social feeling. The same applies to early illnesses, like rickets, that impair the physical, though not the mental development, and may also lead to more or less serious deformities. Among the other diseases of the earliest childhood, those in which the anxiety and care of the persons round the child give him a great sense of his own personal worth without his contributing anything himself are most likely to do injury to social feeling. To this category belong whooping-cough, scarlet fever, encephalitis, and chorea. When they have run their course, often without serious injury, the child will be found to be 'difficult' because, even after he is well, he will still fight to have his pampering continued. Even in cases where physical disabilities remain it will be wise not to refer any deterioration in the child's conduct to these but to leave things alone. I have observed that even in cases where heart trouble and disease of the kidneys had been wrongly diagnosed, the difficulty in training the child did not disappear after the mistake had been discovered and complete health established. Self-love with all its consequences, especially with its lack of social interest, still continued. Anxiety and worry and tears do not help the sick child; they induce him to find an advantage in his illness. It goes without saying that anything injurious to the child that can be corrected should be improved and put right as soon as possible and that in no case should it be assumed that the child will 'outgrow' his faults. Also, in seeking to prevent disease we should try, as far as our means will allow us, to do this without making the child timid and preventing him from getting into contact with other persons.

Burdening a child with things that make too great a demand on his physical or mental resources may easily lead him to take up an attitude opposed to contact with life, by causing him pain or exhaustion. Instruction in art and science should be given in accordance with the degree of the child's capacity to receive it.[1] For the same reason an end must be made to the fanatic insistence of many pedagogues on the explanation of sexual facts. The child ought to receive an answer when he asks or seems to ask about these questions, but one should

[1] cf. Dr. Deutsch, *Klavierunterricht auf individualpsychologischer Grundlage.*

be certain that he is able to assimilate the information that is given him. Early instruction, however, should be given in all cases about the equal worth of the sexes and about the child's own sexual role. Otherwise, as Freud also admits, to-day the child as the result of our backward civilization can get the idea that women have an inferior status. This may easily lead in the case of boys to an arrogant attitude, with all its antisocial consequences, and in the case of girls to the 'masculine protest' described by me in 1912.[1] The results here will be just as bad; doubt with regard to the proper sex will be followed by imperfect preparation for the real sexual role, and this can lead to all kinds of disastrous consequences.

Certain difficulties are caused by the position of the child with reference to the other members of the family. The priority of one of the family in early childhood, whether emphasized or not, often reacts to the disadvantage of one of the other members. With amazing frequency the failures of one child are found beside the successes of the other. The greater activity shown by one may bring about a passive attitude in the other, the success of the one may cause the failure of the other. One can often see the marked effect early failures have on a child's after life. In the same way a preference for one of the children, which is often difficult to avoid, may result in injury to one of the others, since it induces in him an acute feeling of inferiority with all the possible formations of an inferiority complex. The height, the

1 cf. Adler, *Über den nervösen Charakter.*

good looks, or the strength of the one may cast a shadow on the other. In such cases the facts I have brought to light regarding the position of a child in the family constellation are not to be overlooked.

Above all we must rid ourselves of the superstition that the situation within the family is the same for each individual child. We know already that even when all the family have the same environment and the same upbringing the influence of these will be used by the child in a manner that suits the purpose of his creative ability. We shall see how different are the effects of environment on each single child. It seems also to be proved that children of the same family show neither the same genes nor the same phenotypic variations. Even in the case of enzygotic twins there is an ever-increasing doubt as to whether they possess the same physical and psychical constitution.[1]

For a long time now Individual Psychology has been founded on the fact of a congenital physical constitution, but it has proved that the 'psychical constitution' only makes its appearance in the first three to five years of the child's life. The child does this by forming the psychical prototype. This already contains within itself the individual's permanent law of movement and owes its life-pattern to the child's creative energy, which utilizes heredity and the influences of the environment as its material. This conception alone made it possible for me to represent the differences between the members of a family as approximately typical of all families, although

[1] cf. Holub, *Inter. Zeitschr f. Indiv.* (1933).

each individual case has its variations. I consider my problem to have been solved by showing that in the life-pattern of every child there is the imprint of his position in the family succession. This fact throws a vivid light on the problem of the development of character. For if it is correct to say that certain character traits are in harmony with the position of a child in the family sequence, then there is little ground remaining for arguing in favour of the hereditary nature of character, or for deriving it from the anal or from any other zone.

Further, we can easily understand how a child, as the result of his position in the family, acquires a certain definite individuality. The difficulties of an only child are more or less known. Growing up among adults, in most cases looked after with excessive solicitude, with his parents constantly anxious about him, he learns very soon to regard himself as the central figure and to behave accordingly. The sickness or weakness of one of the parents often adds to the difficulty of the situation. Still more frequently marital troubles and divorces produce an atmosphere in the home that has a prejudicial influence on the child's social feeling. As I have pointed out one often finds that there has been a protest, usually of neurotic origin, on the part of the mother against having another child. This protest in most cases is combined with exaggerated care for the only child, and, as a consequence, with his complete enslavement. In later life children like these—with individual variations—are found exhibiting all the gradations between a subjection endured with a secret protest and an excessive craving for sole domination. These are sore spots that begin to bleed and become actively manifest after contact with an exogenous problem. In many cases an attachment to the family that prevents contact with those outside it will prove to be injurious.

When there is more than one child the first-born is in a special situation that is not experienced by any of the other children. For a time he is an only child and as such he receives all his impressions. At varying periods later on he is 'dethroned'. This picturesque expression, which I chose, expresses the change in the situation so exactly that later writers as well, when they do justice to a case like this, for example Freud, cannot deny themselves its use. The period that elapses between birth and this 'dethronement' is of some importance owing to the effect it produces and the elaboration of that effect by the child. If three or more years pass it has its place in the style of life already established and receives a corresponding reaction. As a rule pampered children feel this change as strongly as they do their weaning from the mother's breast. I have to make it clear, however, that even a single year's interval is sufficient to leave visible traces of dethronement on the child's whole life. In this connection we must also take into account the room for movement in life that has already been acquired by the first-born and also the restriction of this that has been caused by the arrival of the second child. It is obvious that a large number of factors have to be taken into consideration if we are to gain a more intimate knowledge of this situation.

231

Above all, too, we have to note that when the interval is not too great the whole process is 'wordless' and is carried through without being expressed in concepts; hence it is not susceptible of correction by later experiences but only by the knowledge of the context gained by Individual Psychology. These wordless impressions, so frequent in early childhood, are otherwise interpreted by Freud and Jung when they come across them at any time. They regard them not as experiences, but, according to their respective views, either as unconscious instincts or as an atavistic social inheritance of the unconscious. Impulses of hate, however, or death wishes, which we find occasionally, are the artificial products of an incorrect training in social feeling. They are well known to us, but we find them only in spoiled children, and they are often directed against the second child. Similar moods and ill-humours are to be found in the children who come later, especially in those who have been pampered. The first-born child, however, when he has been more pampered, has an advantage over the other children on account of his exceptional position, and as a rule he feels his dethronement more acutely. But similar phenomena can be observed in the case of children who come later in the family sequence. These readily give rise to an inferiority complex, and they are sufficient proof that the idea of a somewhat more severe birth-trauma than usual causing failures on the part of the first-born is to be relegated to the region of fables. It is a vague assumption that can be grasped at only by those who have no knowledge of Individual Psychology.

It is also easy to understand that the protest of the first-born against his dethronement very often takes the form of an inclination to recognize any given authority as justified and to side with it. This inclination occasionally gives the first-born child a distinctly 'conservative' character, not in any political sense, but in relation to the facts of everyday life. I found a striking example of this in Theodor Fontane's biography. We need not be accused of splitting hairs when we see the trait of submission to authority in Robespierre's personality also, despite the leading part he played in the Revolution. But, since Individual Psychology is opposed to fixed rules, it ought to be borne in mind that it is not the position in the family sequence that is the decisive factor, but the situation that results from it. Hence the psychical portrait of the first-born may emerge even in a child who comes later in the family succession, if in any way he has his attention more drawn to another who follows him, and if he reacts to that situation. The fact too, that a second-born child can occasionally take up the role of the first-born should not be overlooked, as, for example, in the case where the first-born child is weak-minded and therefore does not come into consideration as part of the normal situation. A good example of this is to be found in the character of Paul Heyse, who took up an almost paternal attitude towards his elder brother and was his teacher's right-hand supporter at school. But in every case we shall find a method of investigation ready to our hand if we make a careful examination of a first-born child's life-pattern and do not forget that the second child presses on his heels. The fact that he is sometimes able to escape from this situation by treating the second child in a fatherly or motherly way is simply a variant of his struggle for the upper hand.

A special problem seems very frequently to arise in connection with first-born children who are followed by a sister at not too great a distance in time. Their social feeling is often subject to serious injuries. The reason is above all that girls in the first seventeen years of their life grow more rapidly than boys, both in body and mind, and therefore press more closely on the heels of the pace-maker. Often, too, the reason is that the older boy not only tries to assert himself on the ground of his natural priority, but endeavours to take a wrong advantage of his masculine role, while the girl, under the influence of our present-day cultural repression, develops a pronounced feeling of inferiority and pushes on vigorously. She thus discloses a more thorough training which often gives her marked traits of greater energy. This is in the case of other girls as well, the prelude to the 'masculine protest'.[1] In the development of girls this can have a vast number of consequences that are both good and bad; they comprise all sorts of human excellencies and shortcomings, not excluding the rejection of love and homosexuality. Freud has made use of this discovery of Individual Psychology and has pressed it into his sexual scheme under the name of the 'castration complex', holding that it is simply the want of the male genital organ that creates that feeling of inferiority whose structure

1 cf. *Über den nervösen Charakter.*

has been discovered by Individual Psychology. Recently, however, he has given some slight indication that he has some interest left for the social side of the problem. The fact that the first-born was almost always regarded as the representative of the family and of its conservative tradition proves once more that intuitive ability is based on experience.

With regard to the impressions under which the second child outlines his self-created law of movement, these are mainly to be found in his having constantly in front of him another child who is not only more advanced in his development, but who also in most cases disputes his claim to equality by keeping the upper hand. These impressions are absent when the gap between their ages is great, and they are all the stronger the narrower that gap is. They can be very oppressive when the second child feels that the first-born cannot be beaten. They almost disappear when the second child is victorious from the start, whether his victory is due to the elder brother's inferiority or to his being less popular. In almost every case, however, one can observe in the second child a more vigorous onward struggle, which shows itself either in his greater energy or in his more impetuous temperament. This may be employed in the furtherance of social feeling or it may result in a failure. We have to find out whether he is mainly under the impression that he is running a race in which his older brother occasionally takes part or whether he does not feel that he is always under full steam. When the sexes are different the rivalry may become keener, in some cases even without doing any essential injury to social feeling. The good looks of one of the children have also to be taken into account. Similarly the coddling of one of two children may be regarded as serious by the other, although the difference of the attention given by the parents may not seem very obvious to an onlooker. If one of them is a pronounced failure, the other may often give promise of being a success, though sometimes this may not prove to be the case when school-life is begun or the period of puberty is reached. If one of the two children receives marked appreciation, the other may easily become a failure. Frequently twins of the same sex are thought to have similar dispositions because they always do the same thing, whether it is good or bad; but in this case we should not overlook the fact that one of them is being towed by the other. In the case of a second child also we have occasion to be surprised at the intuitive ability which outstrips the understanding and is evidently the product of evolution. In the Bible especially the fact of the heaven-storming second son is made wonderfully clear in the story of Jacob and Esau, although we cannot assume that there was any knowledge of this fact. Jacob's longing for the birthright, his wrestling with the angel ('I will not let thee go except thou bless me'), his dream of a ladder reaching to heaven, clearly show the rivalry of the second son. Even those who are not inclined to agree with my view cannot fail to be greatly impressed when they find Jacob's contempt for the first-born in evidence again and again throughout his whole life. The same thing is seen in his persistent wooing of Laban's second daughter, in the slight hope he has of his own first-born and in his giving the greater blessing to the second son of Joseph by the crossing of his hands.

The first-born of two elder daughters in a family turned out to be a wildly rebellious child after the birth of her younger sister when she was three years old. The second daughter 'guessed' that it was to her advantage to become a docile child, and in this way she made herself extremely popular. The more popular she became the more the elder sister raged, and she kept up her furiously protesting attitude until she was quite old. The younger sister, accustomed to being superior in everything, suffered a shock when she was outstripped at school. Her experience at school and, in later years, her meeting with the three life-problems compelled her to establish her retreat from the point that was dangerous for her. At the same time also, as a consequence of her continual fear of defeat, she was forced to construct her inferiority complex in the form of the 'hesitant movement', as I have called it. She was thus no doubt to some extent protected from all defeats. Repeated dreams of arriving too late at a railway station showed the strength of her style of life, which was even present in her dreams to train her for the neglect of opportunities. No human being, however, can find a state of repose in the feeling of inferiority. The struggle for a goal of perfection ordained by evolution for every living being is unresting, and it finds a way of advance either in the direction of social feeling or in a thousand variants opposed to this.

SOCIALLY OBSTRUCTIVE SITUATIONS

The variant urged upon our second-born and found useful after some tentative efforts took the form of a compulsory washing-neurosis. This compulsion to wash her person, her clothes, and her utensils, especially when other people came near her, blocked the way for the fulfilment of her tasks; it was also convenient for killing the time thus left on her hands—and time is the chief enemy of the neurotic. In this way she had guessed without being able to understand that she had surpassed all other persons by the exaggerated exercise of a cultural function which had formerly made her popular. She alone was clean; all other people and everything else were dirty. I do not need to say anything further about her want of social feeling—a want in the case of such an apparently nice child of an excessively pampering mother. Nor need I add that her cure was possible only through a strengthening of her social feeling.

A good deal could be said about the youngest in a family. He, too, finds himself in a fundamentally different situation compared with the other members. He is never the only child, as the eldest is for some time. He has no one following him, however, as all the other children have. Nor has he only one predecessor like the second, but often several. He is in most cases spoiled by elderly parents, and he finds himself in the embarrassing situation of being regarded as the smallest and weakest, and as a rule he is not taken seriously. His lot on the whole, is not unhappy. And he is spurred on daily in his struggle for superiority over those in front of him. In many respects his position is like that of the second child in the

238

family. It is a situation which other children in a different position in the sequence may reach if similar rivalries happen to arise. His strength is often shown in his attempts to excel the rest of his brothers and sisters in the most various degrees of social feeling. His weakness is often seen in his evasion of the direct struggle for superiority—and this seems to be the rule in the case of excessive pampering—and in his seeking to reach his goal on another plane, in another life-pattern, in another calling. When we look into the workings of the psychical life with the eye of the experienced Individual Psychologist we are amazed again and again to perceive how frequently this becomes the fate of the youngest child. If the family consists of business people the youngest becomes a poet or a musician. If the other members of the family are intellectual, the youngest adopts an industrial or a business calling. In this connection the limited opportunities for girls in our very imperfect civilization have to be taken into account.

With regard to the characteristics of the youngest son my references to the Joseph of the Bible have attracted universal attention. I know as well as any one else that Benjamin was Jacob's youngest son. But he was born seventeen years after Joseph and for the most part remained unknown to him. He had no influence on Joseph's development. All the facts are well known— how this lad went among his hard-working brethren dreaming of his future greatness, how bitter their anger was at his dreams of lording it over them and over the world, and of being like God. In addition to this there

239

was certainly also the preference shown for him by his father. But he became the supporting pillar of his family and his tribe, and far more than that—one of the saviours of civilization. In each of his actions and in his works we see the greatness of his social feeling.

The intuition of folk-lore has provided many similar examples. Many others are also to be found in the Bible, e.g. Saul, David, etc. We find them also in the fairy-tales of all ages and peoples. When there is a youngest son in these sagas he is sure to be the victor. Further, we have only to look round on contemporary society to see how often among the very great figures of humanity it is a youngest son who has gained an outstanding position. He frequently counts as well among the most striking failures. This fact can be accounted for again and again by his dependence on a person who has either pampered or neglected him. These are the circumstances out of which he has mistakenly constructed his social inferiority.

This sphere of child-research—the child's position in the family sequence—is by no means completely explored. It shows with compelling clarity how a child utilizes his situation and the impressions derived from it as material for creatively constructing his style of life —his law of movement, and along with this his characteristic traits. It may possibly have become obvious to the student that this leaves little room for the assumption that character traits are hereditary. With regard to the other positions in the family sequence—in so far as they are not simply replicas of those that have been discussed—I have by no means so much to say. Crichton-Miller in London called my attention to the fact that he had found that a third girl following two other girls shows a fairly strong masculine protest. I was able in many cases to confirm the correctness of his discovery. I trace this to the fact that a girl in this position feels, guesses, and even often experiences her parents' disappointment with the birth of another girl, and in some way or other she expresses her dissatisfaction with the female role. It will not be surprising to find in the case of this girl a pretty strong defiant attitude. This shows what Charlotte Bühler professes to have found as a 'natural stage of defiance'. But it can be better understood according to the descriptions of Individual Psychology as an artificial product than as a permanent protest against actual or supposed snubbing.

I have not completed my researches in connection with the development of an only girl among boys and of an only boy among girls. According to what I have noticed till now I expect to find that both will tend to extremes, either in a masculine or in a feminine direction. In the feminine direction when this has been felt in childhood to be more successful, in the masculine when this role seemed to be more worth attaining. In the former case one will find weakness and the need of support to an excessive degree, along with all sorts of petty naughtinesses; in the second case unconcealed craving for mastery and obstinacy, but also occasionally courage and honourable struggle.

CHAPTER XIV

DAY-DREAMS AND NIGHT DREAMS

In our consideration of this subject we enter the realm of fantasy. This function is also the creation of the evolutionary process, and it would be a great mistake to separate it from the unity of the psychical life and from the linking of the psychical life as a whole with the demands of the external world; it would be a still greater mistake to try to put it in opposition to that unity, i.e. to the ego. On the contrary fantasy is a part of the individual style of life, giving it at the same time its character. Regarded as psychical movement it impresses itself on all the other parts of the mental existence in so far as it bears within it the expression of the individual's law of movement. The task given to it is, under certain circumstances, to express itself in mental images, while at other times it lurks in the realm of feelings and emotions, or is imbedded in the individual's attitude to life. Like every other psychical movement it is directed towards the future, since it also moves with the stream towards the goal of perfection. From this point of view it becomes increasingly clear how meaningless it is to

242

see in the movement of fantasy or of its derivatives—day and night dreams—a wish-fulfilment; and how still more futile it is to imagine that any contribution has thereby been made to the understanding of the mechanism of fantasy. Since every psychical expressive form moves from beneath upwards, from a minus to a plus situation, every psychical expressive movement can be described as a wish-fulfilment.

Fantasy, or imagination, more than common sense, makes use of the ability to guess, though by saying that we do not also mean that its guess is 'correct'. Its mechanism consists in its desisting temporarily—in psychosis permanently—from common sense, i.e. from the logic of human communal life, and, from the social feeling existing at present, not content to take with it the next steps in the interests of the community. This is done more easily if the existing social feeling is not particularly strong. But if it is strong enough it may lead the steps of fantasy towards the goal of enriching the community. Invariably, however, the self-originated process of psychical movement is resolved into thoughts, feelings, and a state of preparedness for taking up an attitude towards life. Attitudes are to be recognized as 'correct', 'normal', 'valuable' only when, as in the more notable achievements, they are of service to mankind. A different interpretation of these judgements is logically excluded, though that does not prevent common sense, with its present standards, from rejecting such achievements until a higher level in our knowledge of what is universally good has been reached.

DAY-DREAMS AND NIGHT DREAMS

Every attempt to solve a problem that confronts the individual sets the fantasy to work, since, in seeking a solution, he has to deal with the unknown future. The creative power to which we have assigned the formation of the style of life in childhood is still at work.

The conditioned reflexes, also, in which, with their thousandfold formations, the style of life is active, can only be put to further use as material for its construction.

They are always employed for the creation of some thing completely new; they do not act automatically. But the creative power is exercised along the lines laid down by the style of life that has been formed by the person himself. Thus the guidance of fantasy rests with the style of life. The workings of fantasy give expression to the style of life, whether the individual recognizes this connection or is completely ignorant of it. They can therefore be used as an open door through which we get a glimpse into the workshop of the mind. But if we use the right method we shall always encounter the ego, the personality as a whole; while, if we start with the wrong conception, we shall find what seems to be an antithesis of some kind, such as that between the conscious and the unconscious. Freud, the representative of this incorrect view, by a forced march approaches a better understanding of the problem when he speaks, as he does to-day, of the unconscious in the ego. This, of course, gives the ego quite a different face—a face that Individual Psychology was the first to recognize.

Every great idea and every work of art owe their

DAY-DREAMS AND NIGHT DREAMS

origin to the ceaseless workings of the human spirit that is ever creating afresh. Perhaps most people contribute a small share to these new creations; at the least they can accept them, preserve them, and turn them to account. It is here that the 'conditioned reflexes' may to a large extent have their part to play. For the creative artist they are only building material which his imagination uses to outstrip what has gone before. Artists and geniuses are without doubt the leaders of humanity, and they pay the penalty for their audacity, burning in their own flame which they kindled in childhood. 'I suffered—so I became a poet.' Our improved vision, our better perception of colour, form, and line we owe to the painters. Our more accurate hearing and, along with it, a finer modulation of our vocal organs we have acquired from the musicians. The poets have taught us to speak, feel, and think. The artist himself, in most cases violently spurred on in early childhood, by suffering from all sorts of handicaps—poverty, abnormal sight, or hearing—and as a rule spoiled in some particular way, wrests himself free in his earliest childhood from his severe feeling of inferiority. Fiercely ambitious, he struggles with a too restricted reality in order to broaden it for himself and for others. He is the standard-bearer of an evolution that demands the surmounting of difficulties and raises above the average level the appointed child. Such a child usually suffers in a way suited for the attainment of a lofty goal.

This oppressive but blessed variety of suffering, as we have long ago pointed out, is due to a more marked physical liability to shock, a greater sensitiveness to the influence of external events. These variants very often prove to be inferiorities of the sensory organs in the person himself, or if not in him—since our means of research into the less important variants often fail us— in organ inferiorities inherited from his ancestors. It is in that quarter that we find the clearest traces of such constitutional inferiorities, which often lead to illnesses. They are minus variants which have also been a force behind the progress of humanity.[1] The creative spirit of the child is shown in the games he plays by himself and in the individual manner in which he plays any game. Every game gives scope for the struggle for superiority. Games played in common fit into the impulse to social feeling. Apart from these games in common, solitary occupation both in the case of children and of adults should not be discouraged. Indeed, it should even be encouraged in so far as it allows an outlook on future social enrichment. Owing to the nature of certain activities they can only be exercised and carried out at a distance from other persons; but this by no means detracts from their communal character. Here again imagination is at work, and it is nourished in no small degree by the fine arts. All mental pabulum that cannot be digested ought certainly to be kept away from children's reading until they have reached a certain stage of maturity. Unsuitable literature may either be misunderstood or it may throttle the growing social feeling. To this category belong among others those tales of cruelty that arouse

[1] cf., among others, *Studie über Minderwertigkeit von Organen.*

fear. These have a powerful influence, especially on children whose urinary and sexual systems are stimulated by fear. Again, it is spoilt children who are to be found in this latter category. They are unable to withstand the enticements of the 'pleasure principle'; in their fantasies, and later on in their practices, they create situations that arouse fear for the purpose of inducing sexual excitations. In the course of my examinations of sexual sadists and masochists I have found a similar disastrous concatenation of such circumstances, always combined with a lack of social feeling.

Most of the day-dreams and night dreams of children and of adults lead in the direction given by the goal of superiority, and, up to a certain point, they are freed from the trammels of common sense. It is easy to understand that for the purpose of compensation, as though to maintain the psychical equipoise, the imagination takes precisely that concrete direction which ought to lead to the conquest of a known weakness, although it is never successful along this path. The process is in a certain sense similar to that employed by the child in the creation of his style of life. Fantasy helps to give him an illusory view of increased personal worth at the point where he feels the difficulty, not without spurring him on at the same time to a greater or less degree. Certainly there are plenty of cases where this incitement is lacking, where the fantasy, so to speak, is entirely a matter of compensation. It is obvious that this latter situation is to be regarded as antisocial, although it is devoid of all activity or of any incursion into the external world.

Also when the fantasy, always in accordance with the style of life which leads it, moves contrary to social feeling, it can be recognized as a sign that social feeling has been excluded from the style of life, and it will be a guide for the examiner. This applies to the many cruel day-dreams which occasionally alternate with, or find a substitute in, fantasies about a person's own painful suffering. War-fantasies, dreaming of heroic deeds or the saving of exalted personages as a rule indicate an actual feeling of weakness, and they are replaced in real life by timidity and shyness. Those who perceive here and in similar apparently contrasted expressive forms an ambivalence, a division of consciousness, a double life, are ignorant of the unity of the personality. What is apparently contradictory is deduced simply from an analysis based on the comparison of minus and plus situations and on a mistaken idea of the connection between them. Those who have gained a knowledge of the ceaseless, progressive stream of the mental life will understand that any attempt to characterize correctly a psychical process by a word or a concept is doomed to failure on account of the poverty of our speech, since it is impossible to describe as a static form anything that is in a constant state of flux.

Fantasies frequently occur on the theme of being the child of other parents. These almost certainly point to the dissatisfaction of the child with his own parents. In psychoses, although not in such a pronounced manner in other cases, this fantasy presses reality into the service of a permanent grievance. Whenever a person's

ambition finds reality intolerable he invariably flees to
the magic of fantasy. We do not forget, however, that
when imagination is rightly coupled with social feeling
really great achievements are to be expected; for imagination, by rousing expectant feelings and emotions,
has the same effect as the opening of the throttle of a
motor-car: the activity is increased.

The value of imaginative activity depends above all
on the amount of social feeling with which it is per-
meated. This applies to individuals as well as to the mass.
If we have to deal with a patient who is a definite failure, then we may expect a fantasy that is just as mistaken. The liar, the swindler, the braggart are striking
examples of this. The fool is another. The fantasy is
never at rest, even when it is not condensed into day-
dreams. Like every wish to foresee, the fantasy by being
directed towards a goal of superiority, explores the
future. We must not forget that imagination is a training in the direction of the style of life, whether it makes
its appearance in actual life, in day-dreams and in night
dreams, or creates a work of art. It leads to an exalta-
tion of the person's own individuality, and as it follows
this path it is sometimes more, sometimes less, under
the influence of common sense. Even the dreamer often
knows that he is dreaming. And the person asleep, be
he never so far withdrawn from reality, seldom falls out
of bed. In the dream there is certainly everything which
fantasy employs—wealth, strength, heroic deeds, great
achievements, immortality, etc., hyperbole, metaphor,
simile, symbol. The inciting power of metaphors should

not be overlooked. Despite the want of understanding shown by many of my opponents, metaphors are simply the imaginative disguise of reality and are never identical with it. Their value is undeniable if they are suited to lend additional energy to our life; but we must consider them harmful when they help, by exciting our emotions, to strengthen the antisocial spirit. In every case, however, they serve to evoke and reinforce the emotional tone that is required by the problem which confronts the style of life at the time. They do this when common sense proves inadequate to the occasion or is opposed to the solution demanded by the style of life. This fact will help towards an understanding of the dream.

In order to understand the dream we must first consider sleep. This represents the state of mind in which a dream is possible. Unquestionably sleep is the creation of evolution. It is an independent adjustment which is combined naturally with changes in the physical condition and is brought about by them. Although at present we have only a vague idea of these changes (perhaps the researches of Zondek on the hypophysis have thrown some light on this subject) we may assume that they work in conjunction with the impulse to sleep. Since sleep evidently serves to give rest and recuperation, it also brings all the physical and psychical activities nearer a state of repose. Through waking and sleeping the individual's life-pattern is brought into closer harmony with the alternation of night and day. The mark that differentiates the sleeper from the person who is

awake is the former's concrete distance from the problems of the day.

But sleep is no brother to death. The life-pattern, the
law of movement, continues uninterruptedly. The
sleeper moves, avoids unpleasant positions in bed; he
can be awakened by light and noise; he takes care of a
child sleeping beside him; he carries his daily joys and
sorrows with him. In sleep man is concerned with all
the problems the solution of which will not be interrupted by sleep. An infant's restless movements will
awaken the mother; should we desire it, we wake in the
morning almost regularly at the time required. The
posture of the body in sleep, as I have shown[1] often
gives a good picture of the mental disposition, just as is
the case when the person is awake. The unity of the
psychic life persists even in sleep. Hence we must consider as part of the whole such phenomena as somnam-
bulism, or occasionally suicide during sleep, grinding
the teeth, talking, muscular tension, such as convul-
sive clenching of the hands with subsequent paraesthesia.
We can draw deductions from them, though they must
find further confirmation from other expressive forms.
Emotions also, and moods, are alert in sleep, sometimes
unaccompanied by dreams.

The overwhelming weight of certainty we attach to
things that are seen accounts for the dream's appearing
usually as a visual phenomenon. I have always said
to my students: 'If you are ever in doubt about any
point in your investigations, stop your ears and watch

[1] *Praxis und Theorie der Individualpsycholgie.*

the patient's movement.' Probably every one of us recognizes this greater certainty without putting it into so many words. Is it this greater certainty that the dream is seeking? The dream is further removed than waking life from the daily task; it is dependent on itself alone; it preserves more completely its creative power guided by the style of life; it is more free from the limitations imposed by reality, the law-giver. Does the dream, therefore, give a more vigorous expression to the style of life? The dream is left to the discretion of imagination, which is tethered to the style of life. At other times, also, we find the imagination struggling on behalf of the style of life when a problem confronting the individual is beyond his powers, or when common sense—the individual's social feeling—does not intervene because it does not exist in sufficient strength. Does the dream engage in the same struggle?

We do not mean to follow the example of those who, by ignoring Individual Psychology or by making insinuations against it, wish to take the wind out of its sails. We shall therefore at this point remember Freud, who was the first to attempt to form a scientific theory of dreams. This is a lasting merit that no one can lessen. Nor can any one depreciate certain observations he has made and described as belonging to the 'unconscious'. He seems to have known much more than he understood. It was inevitable, however, that he should go wrong when he forced himself to group all psychical phenomena round the single ruling principle that he recognizes—the sexual libido. This is surely made worse by his fixing his attention only on the mischievous instincts. As I have shown, these arise from the inferiority complex of spoilt children. They are the artificial products of a wrong upbringing and a mistaken self-creation of the child, and they can never lead to an understanding of the psychical structure in its true evolutionary formation. 'If a man could make up his mind to write down all his dreams without distinction and without bias, truthfully and circumstantially, adding to them as a commentary for their explanation all that he could bring from the recollections of his life and from his reading, he would present a notable gift to humanity. But, as mankind is to-day, certainly no one would do this, though even for private and personal encouragement it would be of some value.' Does Freud say this? No, it is Hebel in his *Memoirs*. If this is in brief the conception of the dream I have to add that it depends above all on whether the method adopted will stand a scientific criticism. This was the case to such a small extent with regard to the psycho-analytic method that Freud himself, after numerous changes in his interpretation of dreams, now explains that he never asserted that every dream had a sexual content. Still, this assertion is once more, a step in the right direction.

What Freud calls the 'censor', however, is nothing else than the greater distance from reality that prevails in sleep. It is a purposeful avoidance of social feeling which by its imperfection hinders the individual from solving his problem in the normal way, so that, as in a shock when he is threatened with defeat, he seeks a way to another and easier solution. Here the fantasy under the spell of the style of life ought to give assistance apart from common sense. If one tries to find in this a wish-fulfilment, or, despairingly, a death-wish, he lands in a platitude that tells us nothing about the structure of dreams. For the whole life-process, in whatever way it is regarded, may be described as seeking for a wish-fulfilment.

In my investigations concerning dreams I had two great aids. The first was provided by Freud, with his unacceptable views. I profited by his mistakes. I was never psycho-analysed, and I would have at once rejected any such proposal, because the rigorous acceptance of his doctrine destroys scientific impartiality which in any case is not very great. Still, I am sufficiently acquainted with his theory to be able not only to recognize his mistakes but to predict in the reflected image of a pampered child what his next step will be. I have therefore always recommended my students to make themselves thoroughly acquainted with Freud's doctrine. Freud and his followers are uncommonly fond of describing me in an unmistakably boastful way as one of his disciples, because I had many an argument with him in a psychological group. But I never attended one of his lectures, and when this group was to be sworn in to support the Freudian views I was the first to leave it. No one can deny that I, much more than Freud, have drawn the line sharply between Individual Psychology and psycho-analysis, and that I have never boasted of my former discussions with him. I am sorry that the rise of Individual Psychology and the undoubted influence it has exercised on the transformation of psycho-analysis have been so sorely felt in that quarter. But I know how difficult it is to satisfy spoilt children's conception of the universe. It is in the end not so surprising that after psycho-analysis, without surrendering its fundamental principle, made a steady approach to Individual Psychology, similarities become visible to perplexed minds. It was the manifest effect of indestructible common sense. It will therefore appear to many as though during the last twenty-five years I had unfairly predicted the development of psycho-analysis. I am like the prisoner who never lets his captor free.

My second and much stronger support in the understanding of dreams came from an established fact scientifically confirmed and illumined from many sides—the unity of the personality. The same property of belonging to this unity must characterize the dream. There is regularly a greater distance in dreams than in wakefulness from the influences of reality. This distance is demanded by our style of life, and it characterizes our fantasy during our waking hours as well. But even apart from this, no mental form in the dream should be taken to support any theory that assumes such forms are not identical with those existing in our waking life. The conclusion may be drawn that sleep and the dream-life are variants of our waking life, and also that our waking life is a variant of the other. The supreme law of both life-forms, sleep and wakefulness alike, is this: the ego's sense of worth shall not be allowed to be diminished. Or, to adopt the terminology of Individual Psychology: the struggle for superiority in accordance with the ultimate goal rids the individual of the pressure of his feeling of inferiority. We know the direction the path takes; it deviates to a greater or less extent from social feeling; in other words it is antisocial, it opposes common sense. The ego draws strength from the dream-fantasy in order to solve an imminent problem, since it is lacking in the social feeling the problem demands. It goes without saying that the subjective difficulty of the immediate problem plays the part of a test of social feeling, and it can be so oppressive that even the best of us begin to dream.

We must therefore in the first place make it clear that every dream-state has an exogenous factor. This, of course, means something more than, and something different from, Freud's 'day's residue'. Its significance consists in its being a test and a search for a solution. It includes the 'advance to the goal' and the 'whither' of Individual Psychology in opposition to Freud's regression and the fulfilment of infantile wishes. (The latter again are simply another instance of the unreal world of spoiled children, who want to possess everything and who cannot understand why any of their wishes should remain unfulfilled.) It points to the advancing surge of evolution and shows how each single person represents the path he means to take. It shows his conception of his own nature and of the nature and meaning of life.

Let us turn our attention for a moment from the dream-state. Suppose there is a person faced with a test which he does not feel himself mature enough to meet, on account of his want of social feeling. He takes flight into his imagination. What takes this flight? Of course it is the ego in its style of life. The purpose is to find a solution suited to the style of life. That means, however, with the slight exception of those dreams that have a social value, a solution that does not harmonize with common sense. It is in opposition to social feeling, but it relieves the individual in his distress and doubt, and, more than that, it strengthens him in his style of life, in the value he places on his ego. Sleep, hypnosis when rightly practised, and successful auto-suggestion are simply easier ways to attain this end. The conclusion we have to draw from this is that the dream as the purposeful creation of the style of life seeks to keep at a distance from social feeling and represents that distance. Still, when there is a greater amount of social feeling and when the situations are more menacing one occasionally finds the reverse of this—the conquest of social feeling over the attempts to diverge from it. This again is a case which justifies the assertion of Individual Psychology that the psychical life cannot be reduced to rules and formulae. But it leaves the main thesis unaffected, namely that the dream shows a divergence from social feeling.

Here we meet with an objection which for a long time caused me a great deal of trouble, but to which I am indebted for a profounder insight into the problem of dreams. It is this: if the description of the facts just given is correct, how are we to explain that no one understands his dreams or pays any attention to them, and that in most cases they are forgotten? If we exclude the handful of people who understand something about their dreams, there seems to be a wasteful expenditure of energy in them that we find nowhere else in the economy of the spirit. But here another of our experiences in Individual Psychology comes to our aid. Man knows more than he understands. Is his power of knowing alert in the dream when his understanding is asleep? If this be so, then we must also find evidence of something like this in his waking life. And in fact man understands nothing about his goal, but he pursues it none the less. He understands nothing about his style of life, yet he is continually shackled to it. And if, when he is confronted by a problem, his style of life points to a certain path, like going to a drinking-party or undertaking something that promises to be successful, then thoughts and images always appear on the scene—'securities', as I have called them—for the purpose of making this path attractive to him, although they are not necessarily connected obviously with his goal. When a husband is very dissatisfied with his wife another woman often seems more desirable to him without his making the connection between the two clear to himself, to say nothing of his understanding his implied accusation and revenge. His knowledge of the things that are nearest to him will not become understanding until he has seen them in connection with his style of life and with his immediate problem. Besides, I have already pointed out that fantasy, like the dream, must rid itself of a great deal of common sense. It would accordingly be unreasonable to question the dream about its common sense, as many writers have done, in order to come to the conclusion that dreams are nonsensical. The dream will approach closely to common sense only on the rarest occasions; it will never coincide with it. From this, however, there follows the dream's most important function —*to lead the dreamer away from common sense*—and, as we have shown, the same thing applies to imagination as well. In the dream, therefore, the dreamer commits a self-deception. According to our fundamental principle we are able to add a self-deception which, in the face of a problem for whose solution his social feeling is inadequate, refers him to his style of life so that he may solve his problem in accordance with it; and—since he sets himself free from the reality that demands social interest —images stream in upon him that remind him of his style of life.

Does nothing then remain of the dream when it is over? I believe I have the answer to this most important question. There remains what is always left when one indulges in fantasy—feelings, emotions, and a frame of mind. It follows from the fundamental principle of Individual Psychology—the unity of the personality— that all these function in accordance with the individual's style of life. In one of my first attacks on the Freudian dream-theory in 1918 I asserted on the ground of my experiences that the dream has a forward aim, that it 'puts an edge' on the dreamer for the solution of a problem in his own particular way. Afterwards I was able to complete this view by establishing the fact that it does this, not on the lines of common sense, of social feeling, but 'parabolically', metaphorically, in comparative pictures, somewhat in the manner of a poet when he wishes to arouse feelings and emotions. But this brings us back again to the waking state, and we can add that people completely devoid of the poetic faculty make use of comparisons when they wish to make an impression, if it is only by employing such terms of abuse as 'ass', 'old wife', etc. The teacher does the same when he despairs of explaining anything in simple words.

Two different things happen with comparisons. They are undoubtedly better suited than matter-of-fact expressions to rouse emotions. In the art of poetry and in exalted speech the use of metaphor frankly celebrates its triumph. But as soon as we leave the territory of the arts we see the danger that lurks in the use of comparisons. 'Comparisons are odious' say the common people rightly, and by that they mean that in their use there lies the danger of deception. Accordingly we come to the same conclusion here as before, if we keep in mind the employment of comparison pictures in the dream. They serve to deceive the dreamer and to rouse his emotions; at the same time they create a frame of mind in accordance with the style of life. It may well be that the dream is always preceded by a state of mind that is comparable to doubt—by a problem that requires closer examination. But in that case the dream in conformity with its style of life selects from a thousand possible images only those that are favourable to its aims and

lead to the elimination of practical reason in the interests of the style of life.

We have thus shown that the dreamer's fantasy, just
as it does in other formations, follows in the dream as
well the direction of progress and superiority indicated
by the style of life, even when it requires memory-
images like all our other thinking, feeling, and acting.
Although these memory-images in the life of a pampered
child originate in errors due to pampering, even when at
the same time they express an anticipation of the future,
they should not lead to the erroneous conclusion that
infantile wishes find satisfaction by these means or that
this indicates a regression to a childish stage. Moreover,
we must bear in mind that the style of life selects the
images for its own purpose, so that we can get to understand it from the choice it has made. The assimilation
of the dream-image to the exogenous factor places us
in the position of being able to find the line of movement which the dreamer, in order to do justice to his
law of movement, follows as the result of the reaction
on his style of life to the solution demanded by the problem. The weakness of his position is seen in his calling
to his help comparisons and similes which rouse in a
falsifying manner feelings and emotions, whose true
meaning and worth could not have been tested. These
lead to the strengthening and acceleration of the
movement directed by the style of life, somewhat like
giving more petrol to a running motor. Hence the
unintelligibility of a dream is not a matter of chance,
but a necessity. The same unintelligibility can also

be shown in waking life in many cases when a person wishes to defend his mistakes with far-fetched arguments.

Just as in waking life the dreamer resorts to another means of dispensing with practical reason; he either deals with things merely incidental to his immediate problem or he excludes its principal feature. This process, which one is sometimes inclined to think is extensively employed, is seen to be closely related to the one I described in 1932 in the last volume of the *Zeitschrift für Individualpsychologie* (Hirzel, Leipzig) as a partial, inadequate solution of a problem, and a sign of an inferiority complex. Once again I refuse to lay down rules for the interpretation of dreams, since that requires more artistic inspiration than is needed for the pedantic system of a Beckmesser. The dream tells us nothing more than can be inferred from the other expressive forms as well. It merely enables the observer to recognize how effective the old style of life continues to be, with the result that he will draw the patient's attention to this fact and thus help undoubtedly to convince him. In the interpretation of a dream one should only go so far as to let the patient understand that, like Penelope, he unravels during the night what he has woven during the day. Nor should that style of life be forgotten which, somewhat in the manner of a person who has been hypnotized, compels the fantasy itself in exaggerated, apparent obedience to take the docile path when in the presence of the physician without adopting the attitude that should follow from it. This also is a form of obstinacy which was already practised in a secret fashion in childhood.

Recurring dreams indicate an expression of the law of movement directed by the style of life when confronted by problems felt to be similar in their nature. Short dreams show that a question has been answered concisely and decided upon quickly. Forgotten dreams, it may be conjectured, mean that their emotional tone is strong as opposed to the practical reason, which is just as strong. In order to find a better means of circumventing the latter the intellectual material has to be evaporated so that only emotion and attitude remain. It is frequently found that anxiety dreams reflect heightened anxiety in the face of a defeat, and pleasant dreams a more vigorous 'fiat', or a contrast with the existing situation meant to provoke all the stronger feelings of aversion. Dreams about dead people suggest that the dreamer has not yet finally buried his dead and remains under the dead person's influence. But this has naturally to be corroborated by other expressive forms. Dreams of falling—certainly the commonest of all—indicate that the dreamer is anxious about losing his sense of worth; but at the same time they show by spatial representation that the dreamer is under the delusion that he is 'above'. Flying dreams occur with ambitious people as the precipitate of their struggle for superiority—the struggle to perform something that will exalt the dreamer over all other persons. This dream is frequently accompanied by a falling dream as a warning against an ambitiously risky struggle. A successful land-ing after a dream-fall, often expressed in feeling rather than in thought, may possibly in most cases indicate a sense of security or even a feeling of being predestined, in consequence of which the individual is assured that no harm can come to him. Missing a train or an opportunity can be shown in most cases to be the expression of an established character trait—escaping from a dreaded defeat by arriving too late or by letting an opportunity slip. Dreams about being improperly clothed followed by fright on that account can be mostly traced back to the fear of being detected in an imperfection. Kinaesthetic, visual, and acoustic tendencies are frequently expressed in dreams; still they are always combined with a definite attitude to an immediate problem. On rare occasions, as individual instances show, the solution of the problem can even be assisted by such dreams. When the dreamer plays the part of a spectator it is almost certain that in waking life he would willingly be satisfied with the role of onlooker. Sexual dreams point in different directions. Sometimes they show a comparatively inadequate training for sexual intercourse; at other times they reveal a retreat from a partner and a withdrawal upon oneself. With regard to homosexual dreams I have strongly enough emphasized the training against the other sex. There is nothing here in the nature of an inborn tendency. Dreams of cruelty in which the individual takes an active part betoken rage and a craving for revenge. The same applies to dreams of pollution. Children who wet their beds often dream that they are urinating at the proper place. In this rather cowardly fashion they find it easy to express their grievance and their revenge at the feeling of being neglected. There are a large number of interpreted dreams in my books and writings; for that reason I shall refrain from giving definite examples here. The following dream can be taken as an illustration of the connection with the style of life:

A husband, the father of two children, quarrelled a great deal with his wife. This state of strife was fanned into flame by both of them. The husband knew that his wife had not married him for love. He had been to begin with a spoilt child, but he had afterwards been dethroned by another child. He had, however, learned in a hard school to control his angry outbursts. He even went so far as often to make too protracted attempts in a difficult situation to effect a peaceful reconciliation with his opponents, though these attempts, as may be imagined, were seldom successful. In his relations with his wife his attitude was a mixture of opposites. Sometimes he would wait patiently, attempting to create an atmosphere of affection and confidence, at other times he would have sudden outbursts of fury, when he relapsed into a feeling of inferiority and was at his wit's end. His wife completely misunderstood this situation. The husband doted on his two boys with unusual affection, and they on their part responded to him. The mother, whose formal coolness naturally made her incapable of rivalling her husband in the children's affections, gradually lost touch with them. This seemed to the man like neglect of the children and he often reproached his wife on that account. Their marital relations continued under difficulties, but they were both determined to avoid having any more children. For a long time this was the situation between the two partners: the husband, who could only recognize love in strong emotions, felt himself defrauded of his conjugal rights, while the wife, frigid by the very nature of her style of life and lacking the desired warmth of feeling for her husband or children, made futile attempts to continue the marriage. One night the husband dreamed of bleeding female bodies that were being flung about unfeelingly. My conversation with him led him to the recollection of a scene in a dissecting room where a medical friend had taken him. But it was easy to see—and this was confirmed by the man himself—that the act of childbirth, which he had witnessed on two occasions, had affected him deeply. The interpretation was: 'I do not intend to stand another confinement of my wife.'

Another dream ran: 'It seemed to me as though I were searching for my third child, who had either been lost or kidnapped. I was terribly anxious. All my efforts and exertions proved fruitless.' As the man did not have a third child, it was clear that he was continually in dread that a third child would be in the greatest danger on account of his wife's inability to look after his children. The dream occurred shortly after the kidnapping of the Lindbergh baby and it showed an exogenous shock-problem corresponding to the patient's style of life and his meaning—rupture of relations with a person who has no warm feeling, and, as a part of this intention, the determination to have no more children.

In this dream there is an exaggerated emphasis on his wife's neglect of the children, but it also tends in the same direction as the first dream—towards excessive dread of the act of child-bearing.

The patient came to be treated for impotence. Further traces led back into his childhood. He had learned then, after fairly long and strenuous efforts, to indemnify himself against being slighted by a rejection of the person considered unfeeling, and at the same time also he found it intolerable that his mother should bear any more children. We cannot fail to recognize this man's character-traits and see them in their relation to one another—the main feature of his style of life, his choice of certain images, his self-deception and his auto-intoxication with similes far removed from practical reason that give new energy and enhanced strength to his style of life, his retreat from the problems of life due to the permanent effects of a shock and obtained surreptitiously rather than worked out in accordance with common sense, and his imperfect half-solution of his problem corresponding to his weakness.

If a few words ought to be added about what is described as Freud's dream-symbolism, I can at any rate say this from my experience: it is true that from time immemorial man has shown a tendency to make jocular comparisons between the facts of everyday life and other activities and objects besides the sexual. That has always been done round inn tables and in making smutty jokes. The attraction of these jocular comparisons certainly

lies, to a great extent, not only in the desire to belittle
serious things and in the passion for joking and brag-
ging, but also in the wish to give play to the emotional
accent implied in the symbol. It does not require much
intelligence to understand these everyday symbols which
are to be found in folk-lore and in street-ballads. It is
more important to understand that they certainly occur
in dreams for a definite purpose, which has first of all
to be discovered.

It is to Freud's credit that he has drawn attention to
this. But to explain everything that is not understood as
a sexual symbol and then to discover that everything
springs from the sexual libido will not stand intelligent
criticism. The so-called 'corroborative experiences' with
hypnotized persons, too, supply very weak proofs. It
was first of all suggested to these persons that they *should*
dream of sexual scenes and from their subsequent com-
munications it was then found that they had dreamed in
Freudian symbols. At the most this choice of familiar
symbols instead of undisguised sexual expressions shows
a natural sense of modesty. Besides, it is difficult to-day
for the follower of Freud to get any one to subject himself to such hypnotic experiments who is not acquainted
with the Freudian theory. This is quite apart from the fact
that the 'Freudian symbolism' has considerably enriched
the popular vocabulary and has quite destroyed any frank-
ness in discussing these otherwise very harmless subjects.
One can quite often observe in the case of patients
who have been under psycho-analytic treatment that
they make an extensive use of the Freudian symbolism.

CHAPTER XV

THE MEANING OF LIFE

The question as to the purport of life has worth and meaning only if we keep in view the related system of man and the cosmos. When we do this it is easy to see that the cosmos in this relationship possesses a formative power. The cosmos is, so to speak, the father of everything that lives, and all life is engaged in a constant struggle to satisfy its demands. This does not mean that there exists in it an impulse which would be capable later of bringing everything in life to completion and that only needs to unfold itself, but rather that there is something inherent which is part and parcel of life itself, a struggle, an urge, a self-development, a something without which life cannot be conceived. To live means to develop oneself. The human spirit is only too well accustomed to reduce everything that is in flux to a form, to consider it not as movement but as frozen movement—movement that has become form. We Individual Psychologists have for some time been on the way to resolve into movement that which we conceive of as form. Every one knows that the completed

269

individual man springs from a single cell; but it should also be clearly understood that in this cell are the ingredients necessary for his development. How life came to this earth is a doubtful question; perhaps we shall never find a final answer to it.

The development of living things from a diminutive living unity could only take place with the sanction of the cosmic influence. In regard to this we may think as Smuts has done in his ingenious work, *Wholeness and Evolution*; we may assume that life exists in inorganic matter as well—an idea suggested to us by modern physical science, when it shows us how the electrons revolve about the proton. Whether this view will turn out to be right in the end we do not know. Certain it is that our conception of life cannot be doubted any longer, and that in it a movement is implicit which strives towards self-preservation, towards propagation, and towards contact with the external world—a contact that must be victorious if life is not to succumb. In the light that Darwin has shed we can understand the selection of all those species that can turn to advantage the demands of the external world. Lamarck's view, which is more akin to our own, gives us proofs of the creative energy that is inherent in every form of life. The universal fact of the creative evolution of all living things can teach us that a goal is appointed for the line of development in every species—the goal of perfection, of active adaptation to the cosmic demands.

We have to start from this path of development, of continuous, active adaptation to the demands of the external world, if we wish to understand in what direction life proceeds and moves. We have to realize that we are dealing here with something primordial, with something that has clung to primeval life. It is always a question of overcoming, of the stability of the individual and the human race; it is always a question of promoting a favourable relation between the individual and the external world. This compulsion to carry out a better adaptation can never come to an end. I developed this idea as early as 1902[1] and drew pointed attention to the fact that this 'truth' is a constant menace to any failure in this active adaptation, and that it is to this same failure that we can attribute the extermination of peoples, families, individuals, and animal and vegetable species.

When I speak of active adaptation I exclude the fanciful ideas that link this adaptation with the present-day situation, or with the death of everything living. It is a question rather of adaptation *sub specie aeternitatis*, for only that physical and psychical development is 'right' which can be reckoned as right for the uttermost future. Moreover, the idea of an active adaptation means that body and mind, as well as the whole of organized life, have to strive to attain the ultimate adaptation, the mastery of all the advantages and disadvantages ordained by the cosmos. Apparent compromises which last for a limited period succumb sooner or later beneath the weight of the truth.

We are in the midst of the stream of evolution, but

[1] cf. *Heilen und Bilden.*

we notice this as little as we do the spinning of the earth on its axis. One of the conditions in this cosmic connection in which the individual's life is a part is the struggle for a victorious assimilation with the external world. Even if there should be any doubt about the existence of this struggle at the beginning of life, the billions of years that have elapsed make it clear that the struggle for perfection is an inborn actuality existing in every person. And this consideration can show something else as well. None of us knows which is the only right path to follow. Mankind has made many attempts to imagine this final goal of human evolution. The belief that the cosmos ought to have an interest in the preservation of life is scarcely more than a pious hope. As such, however, it can be used, and has been used, in religion, morals, and ethics as a powerful motive force for the furtherance of human welfare. The worship, too, of a fetish, of a lizard, of a phallus as a fetish in a prehistoric tribe does not seem to be scientifically justifiable. Still we should not overlook the fact that this primitive conception of the universe has furthered communal life, the social feeling of humanity, since every one who was under the spell of the same religious fervour was regarded as a brother, as taboo, and was accorded the protection of the chief tribe.

The best conception hitherto gained for the elevation of humanity is the idea of God.[1] There can be no question that the idea of God really includes within it as a

[1] cf. Jahn und Adler, *Religion und Individualpsychologie* (Verlag Dr. Passer, Vienna, 1933).

goal the movement towards perfection, and that, as a concrete goal, it best corresponds to the obscure yearning of human beings to reach perfection. Certainly it seems to me that every one conceives of God in a different way. There are no doubt conceptions of God that from the very start fall far short of the principle of perfection; but of its purest form we can say—here the presentation of the goal of perfection has been successful. The primal energy which was so effective in establishing regulative religious goals was none other than that of social feeling. This was meant to bind human beings more closely to one another. It must be regarded as the heritage of evolution, as the result of the upward struggle in the evolutionary urge. An immense number of attempts have been made to represent this goal of perfection. We Individual Psychologists, especially those of us who are physicians and have to deal with failures, with persons who suffer from a neurosis or a psychosis, with delinquents, drunkards, etc., see the goal of superiority in them as well; but it leads in a direction so opposed to reason that we are unable to recognize in it a proper goal of perfection. When, for example, a person seeks to make his goal concrete by wishing to domineer over others, this goal of perfection seems to us to be unfitted to guide either the individual or the mass of men, because it could not be the task of every one. The individual would be compelled to oppose the urge of evolution, to violate reality, and to protect himself in utter fear against the truth and against those who follow it. Dependence on other persons is taken by many as their goal of perfection; this too seems to us to be opposed to reason. Some find their goal in leaving the problems of life unsolved, in order to avoid defeats that would otherwise be inevitable and would be contrary to their goal of perfection. This goal, too, seems to us to be thoroughly unsuitable, although it appears to be acceptable to many people.

When we enlarge our outlook and ask what has happened to those forms of life that have chosen a faulty goal of perfection, failing in active adaptation because they have followed the wrong path, and missing the path of universal progress, we find our answer in the extinction of species, races, tribes, families, and thousands of individual persons that have left no trace behind them. They teach us how necessary it is for every person to find a goal that is even tolerably right. It goes without saying that in our day as well the goal of perfection gives the direction for the development of the individual's whole personality, for all his expressive forms, for his seeing, his thinking, his emotions, his view of the universe. And it is just as clear and as intelligible for every Individual Psychologist that a line that deviates to any extent from the truth must lead to the injury of the person who follows it, if not to his overthrow. It would really be a fortunate discovery if we knew more about the direction we have to take, since, after all, we are immersed in the stream of evolution and are compelled to follow its course. Here, too, Individual Psychology has achieved a great deal, just as it has done with the establishment of the universal struggle for perfection.

As the result of its manifold experience it is in the position of understanding in a certain measure the direction in which an ideal perfection is to be found, and indeed it has shown this direction by establishing the norm of *social feeling*.

Social feeling means above all a struggle for a communal form that must be thought of as eternally applicable, such as, say, could be thought of when humanity has attained its goal of perfection. It is not a question of any present-day community or society, or of political or religious forms. On the contrary, the goal that is best suited for perfection must be a goal that stands for an ideal society amongst all mankind, the ultimate fulfilment of evolution. It will, of course, be asked: How do I know that? Certainly not from my immediate experience, and I must admit that those who find an element of metaphysics in Individual Psychology are quite right. To some this is a matter for praise, others condemn it. Unfortunately there are many people who have a wrong idea of metaphysics; they wish to exclude from human life all that they cannot grasp directly. By doing this we would limit the potential development of every new idea. Immediate experiences never result in anything new; that is given only with the comprehensive idea that connects these facts. This new idea may be called speculative or transcendental, but there is no science that does not end in metaphysics. I see no reason to be afraid of metaphysics; it has had a great influence on human life and development. We are not blessed with the possession of absolute truth; on that account we are compelled to form theories for ourselves about our future, about the result of our actions, etc. Our idea of social feeling as the final form of humanity—of an imagined state in which all the problems of life are solved and all our relations to the external world rightly adjusted—is a regulative ideal, a goal that gives us our direction. This goal of perfection must bear within it the goal of an ideal community, because all that we value in life, all that endures and continues to endure, is eternally the product of this social feeling.

In the preceding chapters I have described the facts, the results, and the defects of our present-day social feeling in the individual and in the mass, and I have done my best in the interests of the knowledge of humanity and of the science of character to set forth my experiences and to show how it was possible to throw light on the law of movement in the individual and in the mass as well as on their mistakes. In Individual Psychology all irrefutable facts of experience are looked at and understood from this point of view, and its scientific system has been developed under the pressure of these experiential facts. The results obtained do not contradict one another and they are confirmed by common sense. Individual Psychology has done all that is necessary to satisfy the demands of a rigorous scientific doctrine. It has brought forward an immense number of immediate experiences and arranged them in a system that accommodates itself to these experiences and does not contradict them; it has also supplied the trained ability to guess in accordance with common sense—an

ability that is equal to seeing experiences in their connection with the system. This ability is all the more
necessary since each case has a different complexion
from any other and always gives occasion for fresh efforts
at artistic guessing. If I am venturing now to maintain
the right of Individual Psychology to be accepted as a
view of the universe, since I use it for the purpose of
explaining the meaning of life, I have to exclude all
moral and religious conceptions that judge between virtue and vice. I do this although I have been convinced
for a long time that both ethics and religion as well as
political movements have continually aimed at doing
justice to the meaning of life and that they have developed under the pressure of social feeling, which is an
absolute truth. The position of Individual Psychology
with reference to them is determined by its scientific
knowledge, and certainly also by its more direct effort
to develop social feeling as knowledge more effectively.
According to this position every tendency should be
reckoned as justified whose direction gives undeniable
proof that it is guided by the goal of universal welfare.
Every tenet should be held to be wrong if it is opposed
to this standpoint or is vitiated by the query of Cain:
'Am I my brother's keeper?'

Supported by the facts already established, I may in
a brief attempt make clear that when we enter life we
only find what our ancestors have completed as their
contribution to evolution and the higher development
of all mankind. This one fact alone should show us how
life continues to progress, how we get nearer to a state

in which larger contributions and greater co-operation are possible, and in which every single person in fuller measure than before represents a part of the whole. For this state all forms of social movements are tentative and act as preparations; and only those will last that tend in the direction of an ideal society. While this task has called forth immense and manifold human powers, it has in many respects remained unfinished, and has indeed sometimes proved to have been wrongly carried out. But that is only a sign that humanity in its onward movement along the path of evolution finds 'absolute truth' always beyond its grasp, although it is always capable of getting nearer to it. It shows, too, that there is an immense number of social achievements that last only for a certain period, and during a certain situation, and that even prove harmful after a lapse of time. The only thing that can save us from being crucified on a harmful fiction or from clinging to a scheme of life based on a harmful fiction is the guiding star of universal welfare; under its lead we shall be more able to find the path without suffering any setbacks.

The general welfare and the higher development of humanity are based on the eternally imperishable contributions of our forefathers. Their spirit lives for ever. It is immortal as others are in their children. The continuance of the human species rests on both these factors. Whether or not mankind knows this is immaterial. It is the facts that count. The question as to the right path seems to me to be answered, although we are often groping in the dark. We have no desire to make a final decision; but this one thing we can say: A movement of the individual or of the mass can only be counted worthy by us if it creates values for eternity, for the higher development of the whole of humanity. One ought not to cite one's own stupidity or that of other people as a refutation of this argument. It is obvious that we are concerned not with the possession of truth, but with the struggle for it.

This fact becomes more impressive, not to say more obvious, if we ask: What has happened to those people who have contributed nothing to the general welfare? The answer is: They have disappeared completely. Nothing remains of them; they are quenched body and soul. The earth has swallowed them. It has happened with them as it did with animal species that have become extinct because they were unable to get into harmony with cosmic facts. Surely there is a secret ordinance here. It is as though the questioning cosmos had given the command: 'Away with you! You have not grasped the meaning of life. You cannot endure into the future!'

This is certainly a cruel law. It can only be compared to the terrible deities of ancient peoples and the idea of taboo which threatened with destruction all who set themselves against the community. Thus the emphasis is laid on the permanence, the eternal survival of the contributions of human beings who have achieved something for the general good. We are certainly prudent enough not to assume that we possessed the open sesame for this, and were able to say precisely in every case what is eternally of value and what is not. We are convinced that we can make mistakes, that only a very careful, objective investigation can decide any issue, and that often a decision must be left to the course of events. We have perhaps taken a great step in advance in being able to avoid anything that does not contribute to the community.

Our social feeling to-day has a much wider range than before. Without having understood what we were doing we seek to establish by various and often wrong methods a harmony with the well-being of humanity in education, in the conduct of the individual and of the mass, in religion, science, and politics. Naturally the person who possesses the most social feeling is nearest the comprehension of this future harmony. And on the whole this basic social principle instead of casting down the stumblers has opened up a way for their support.

If we look at our present-day civilized life and keep firmly in mind the fact that the child has already unchangeably settled the extent of his social feeling for his whole life, if there has been no further intervention that would lead to its improvement, then our attention is drawn to certain general conditions whose influence can do great injury to the development of the child's social feeling. Thus there is the fact of war and its glorification in school-teaching. Involuntarily the child whose social feeling is perhaps immature and weak accommodates himself to a world in which it is possible to compel men to fight against machines and poison gas. He is made to feel that it is an honourable thing to kill as many of his fellow beings as he can, although they also would certainly be of value for the future of humanity. The same result follows, though in a lesser degree, from the death penalty; nor are its injurious effects on the childish spirit very much bettered by the consideration that it is a question not so much of fellow creatures as of a person whose hand has been lifted against them. In the case of children with slight inclination for co-operation even the abrupt experience of the death problem can put a swift end to their social feeling. In a similar way girls are endangered when the thoughtlessness of those around them makes them dread the problems of love, procreation, and birth. The unsolved financial problem proves an excessive burden for the developing social feeling. Suicide, crime; bad treatment of old people, cripples, or beggars; prejudices and unjust dealing with persons, employees, races, and religious communities; the maltreatment of the feeble and of children; marital quarrels, and any kind of attempt to give women an inferior position, and much else—ostentatious display of wealth and birth, cliques and their effects on all the strata of society—all these, along with pampering and the neglect of children, put an early end to the development into a fellow being. In our day, in addition to the restoring of the child to his place in co-operation, the only thing that helps against such dangers is the properly timed explanation of the fact that so far we have only reached a comparatively low level of social feeling, and that a real fellow creature must see it his task to co-operate for the amelioration of this wrong state of things for the good of the community; and further that he must not expect this amelioration to be brought about by some mythical tendency to evolve, or through the efforts of other people. Attempts even when made with the best intentions, to attain a higher development through the intensifying of one of these evils, by war, or by the death penalty, or by racial and religious hate, will invariably lead to a lowering of the social feeling in the next generation, and along with that an essential worsening of the other evils. It is interesting, too, to note that such hates and persecutions almost always cause a vulgarizing of life, comradeship, and love-relationships—a fact in which one can clearly see the depreciation of social feeling.

In the foregoing chapters I have supplied enough material to let the reader understand that he is dealing here with a scientific exposition when I emphasize the fact that the individual's proper development can only progress if he lives and strives as a part of the whole. The shallow objections of individualistic systems have no meaning as against this view. I could go still further and show how all our functions are calculated to bind the single individual to the community, and not to destroy the fellowship of man with man. The act of seeing means to receive and make fruitful all that falls on the retina. This is not simply a physiological process; it shows that man is part of a whole that gives and takes. In seeing, hearing, and speaking we bind ourselves to one another. Man only sees, hears, and speaks rightly when he is linked to others by his interest in the external world. His reason, his common sense, forms the basis of his control of co-operation, of absolute truth, and aims at eternal rightness. Our aesthetic sense and views—perhaps the strongest powers that impel to great achievements—have an eternal value only when they lead to the well-being of humanity in the direction of the evolutionary stream. All our bodily and mental functions are rightly, normally, and healthily developed in so far as they are imbued with sufficient social feeling and are fitted for co-operation.

When we speak of virtue we mean that a person plays his part; when we speak of vice we mean that he interferes with co-operation. I can, moreover, point out that all that constitutes a failure is so because it obstructs social feeling, whether children, neurotics, criminals, or suicides are in question. In every case it can be seen that a contribution is lacking. No isolated persons are to be found in the whole history of humanity. The evolution of humanity was only possible because mankind was a community, and in striving for perfection it has striven for an ideal community. This fact finds expression in a person's every movement and function, whether he has found the right direction or not in the stream of evolution, which is characterized by the social ideal. The reason is that man is inviolably guided, hindered, punished, praised, and advanced by the social ideal, and thus each separate individual is not only responsible for every deviation from it, but has also to expiate it. This is a harsh, even a cruel law. Those who have already developed a strong social feeling ceaselessly endeavour to alleviate the rigours of this law for those who have gone in a wrong direction, just as if they knew that this was a human being who had missed the path for reasons that Individual Psychology was the first to point out. If the person understood how in evading the demands of evolution he had gone astray, then he would give up his present course and join the general mass of humanity.

All the problems of human life demand, as I have said, capacity for co-operation and preparation for it— the visible sign of social feeling. In this disposition courage and happiness are included, and they are to be found nowhere else.

All character traits reveal the degree of social feeling; they follow a path which in the meaning of the individual leads to the goal of superiority. They are guiding-lines interwoven with the style of life, which has formed them and again and again brings them to light. Our speech is too inadequate to express the creations of the psychic life in a single word. So when we say 'character-traits' we thereby overlook the manifoldness which is concealed by this expression. Hence for those who depend on words, contradictions gleam through them in such a way that the unity of the psychic life never becomes clear.

Perhaps what will bring the strongest conviction to many is the simple fact that everything we call a mistake shows a want of social feeling. All errors in childhood and in adult life, all faulty character traits in the family, at school, in life, in relationships with other persons, in work, and in love originate in a lack of social feeling.

They may be temporary or permanent, and they vary in a thousand ways.

A careful consideration of individual and collective existence, both past and present, shows us the struggle of mankind for a stronger social feeling. One can scarcely fail to see that humanity is conscious of this problem and is impressed by it. Our present-day burdens are the result of the lack of a thorough social education. It is the pent-up social feeling in us that urges us to reach a higher stage and to rid ourselves of the errors that mark our public life and our own personality. This social feeling exists within us and endeavours to carry out its purpose; it does not seem strong enough to hold its own against all opposing forces. The justified expectation persists that in a far-off age, if mankind is given enough time, the power of social feeling will triumph over all that opposes it. Then it will be as natural to man as breathing. For the present the only alternative is to understand and to teach that this will inevitably happen.

ADDENDUM

CONSULTANT AND PATIENT

Our fundamental principle of the unity of the style of life fashioned in the earliest childhood was already known to me when I began my labours, although I did not understand it, and it enabled me to assume at once that the person who comes for advice reveals his personality the moment he appears, without knowing very much about it. For the patient the consultation is a social problem. Every encounter of one person with another is a problem of that kind. Everyone will introduce himself according to his law of movement. The expert can often tell something of the patient's social feeling at the first glance. Dissimulation is of little use with an experienced Individual Psychologist. The patient expects a good deal of social feeling from his adviser. Since experience has taught us not to expect much social interest from the patient, one will not demand very much. There are two considerations that give us essential help in this connection. The first is that as a rule the general level of social feeling is not high; the second is that we have usually to deal with people who have been pampered as children, and who in their later years cannot free themselves from their unreal world. It would not be very surprising if many of my readers have accepted without a shock the fact that people ask: 'Why should I love my neighbour?' After all Cain put a similar question.

The glance, the gait, the vigour or weakness of the patient's approach can reveal a great deal. Much may be missed if one makes it a rule to indicate, say, a particular seat—a sofa—or to keep strictly to a special hour. The first interview should be a test by its being entirely unconstrained. Even the way of shaking hands may suggest a definite problem. One often sees pampered persons leaning against something and children clinging to their mother. But, just as with everything that constitutes a problem for the consultant's ability to guess, so in these cases also one should avoid rigorous rules and make a close examination. It is preferable to keep one's views to oneself, so that later on, after the case has been understood, they may be used in a suitable way without injuring the patient's hypersensitiveness, which is always in evidence. Occasionally one should tell the patient to sit anywhere he likes, without indicating any particular seat. The distance from the doctor or the consultant reveals—precisely as it does in the case of school-children—a good deal about the patient's nature. Further, it is important that the 'popular' psychology that is the rage in such consultations, and even in social gatherings, should be rigorously forbidden, and that at the beginning of the treatment strictly technical answers to the questions of the patient or his relatives should be avoided. The Individual Psychologist should not forget that, leaving out of account his own trained ability to guess, he has also to bring proof to others who have not had his experience. To the parents and relatives of the patient the consultant should never appear to be taking up an attitude of doubt. He should rather describe the case as worth consideration and not hopeless, even when he is not inclined to undertake it himself, unless weighty reasons in an absolutely hopeless case demand the telling of the truth. I see an advantage in not interrupting the patient's movements. Let him get up, come and go, or smoke as he likes. I have even occasionally given my patients the opportunity of going to sleep in my presence —a suggestion on their part made for the purpose of making my task more difficult. Such an attitude was just as significant a language for me as if they had expressed themselves in words that showed their opposition. A patient's sidelong glance clearly indicates his slight inclination to take part in the common task that links the patient to the doctor. This disinclination to co-operation can be strikingly shown in another way, when the patient says little or nothing, when he beats about the bush, or when he prevents the doctor from speaking by his incessant talking. The Individual Psychologist, unlike other psychotherapeutists, will avoid being sleepy, or going to sleep or yawning, showing a want of interest in the patient, using harsh words, giving premature advice, letting himself be looked upon as the last resort, being unpunctual, getting into a dispute, or declaring that there is no prospect of a cure. In the latter case, when the difficulties are too great, the course recommended is to explain that one is unable to deal with the case and to refer the patient to others who may be more capable. Any attempt at assuming an authoritative manner prepares the way for a failure, and all boasting is an obstacle to the cure. From the very beginning of the treatment the consultant must try to impress on the patient that the responsibility for his cure rests in his own hands. For as the English proverb very rightly says: 'You can take a horse to the water, but you can't make him drink.'

It should be a strict rule to consider the success of the treatment and the cure as due not to the consultant but to the patient. The adviser can only point out the mistakes, it is the patient who must make the truth living. Since, as we have seen, all cases of failure are due to a want of co-operation, advantage should be taken from the start of every means by which the patient's co-operation with the consultant can be increased. Obviously this is only possible when the patient can trust his adviser. Consequently this work in common is of supreme importance as the first serious attempt made in a scientific spirit to lift the social feeling to a higher level. Among other things the consultant must strictly avoid calling into existence—especially by insisting on suppressed sexual components—that psychic current which Freud has called the positive transference. This is frankly demanded in the psycho-analytic cure, and it is also used by other consultants when there is a permanent

T   289

feeling of inferiority and when the patient has very little faith in his adviser, but it only adds a new problem to the treatment. This artificially created condition has, at the best, to be made to disappear. If the patient, who is almost always a spoilt child or an adult craving to be pampered, has learned to take full responsibility for his behaviour, the consultant will easily avoid leading him into that snare which seems to promise an easy and immediate satisfaction of his unfulfilled desires. Since on the whole every unfulfilled wish appears to be a repression to spoilt persons, I should like to say once more here that Individual Psychology demands the repression of neither justifiable nor unjustifiable wishes. It does teach, however, that unjustifiable wishes must be recognized as being opposed to social feeling, and that they can be made to disappear not by suppression but by an addition to social interest. On one occasion I was actually menaced by a weakly man who suffered from dementia praecox, and who was completely cured by me after he had been declared incurable three years before I began to treat him. I already knew at that time that he certainly expected to be given up and rejected by me as well. Such was the fate that had hovered before him ever since he was a child. For three months he remained silent during the treatment. I made this the occasion of giving him cautious explanations in so far as I knew the facts of his life. I recognized, too, an inclination to obstruct me in his silence and in other actions with a similar tendency, and I saw that I was face to face with the culmination of his attitude towards me when he lifted his hand to strike me. I instantly resolved not to defend myself. A further attack followed during which a window was smashed. In the friendliest way I bound up a wound in the patient's hand that was bleeding slightly. (In this case, however, I do not advise my friends to make a rule of such treatment.) When I was completely assured of success in my treatment of this man I asked him: 'Well, what do you think? How are we both going to succeed in curing you?' The answer I received ought to make a very strong impression in interested circles. It has taught me to smile at all the attacks of less-equipped psychologists and psychiatrists who continue to tilt against windmills. He replied: 'That's quite simple. I had lost all courage to live. In our consultations I have found it again.' All who have recognized the simple truth taught by Individual Psychology—that courage is an aspect of social feeling—will understand this man's transformation.

The patient must in any case get the conviction that he is absolutely free with regard to the treatment. He can do or leave undone anything he likes. One should only avoid giving the impression that the patient will begin to get rid of his symptoms even at the very beginning of the treatment. The relatives of an epileptic were told by another adviser at the first consultation that if the patient were left alone he would have no more attacks. The result was that on the first day he had a violent attack on the street and fractured his lower jaw. Another case was less tragic. A youth came to a psychiatrist to be treated for kleptomania, and he carried off

291

the doctor's umbrella after the first consultation.

I will make another recommendation. The doctor should bind himself not to speak to any one else of his conversations with the patient—and he should keep his word. On the other hand the patient should be left absolutely free to tell anything he thinks fit. Certainly one runs the risk here of a patient's using the doctor's explanations to slip into the 'popular' psychology in company. ('What they've learned yesterday they want to teach to-day. What a swift evacuation they must surely have!'); but a friendly talk can take the edge off that. Or there may follow complaints about the patient's family. These must also be anticipated in order to make it plain to the patient beforehand that his relatives are to blame only so long as he makes them blameworthy by his conduct, and that they will immediately be blameless as soon as he feels himself well. Further, it must be pointed out to him that one cannot expect more knowledge from the patient's relatives than he himself possesses and that he has on his own responsibility used the influences of his environment as material for constructing his own style of life. It is also as well to remind him that his parents in the event of their being at fault can appeal to the mistakes of their parents, and so on through the generations; so that for this reason there can be no blame in his sense of the word.

It seems to me important that the patient should not get the idea that the work of an Individual Psychologist is meant to add to his own gain and glory. Keenness to secure patients can only cause harm. This is true also of depreciatory or perhaps spiteful remarks about other consultants.

One example of this will be enough. A man came to me to be cured of nervous exhaustion, which proved to be the result of a fear of being defeated. He informed me that he had been recommended to consult another psychiatrist whom he wished to visit. I gave him the address. On the following day he came to me and told me of his visit. The psychiatrist, after hearing the history of his case, advised him to take the cold-water cure. The patient told him that he had already tried this cure five times without success. The physician advised him to try it for the sixth time in a well-conducted establishment which he particularly recommended. The patient replied that he had been there twice and had been treated unsuccessfully with the water cure. He added that he wanted to come to me for treatment. The psychiatrist advised him against this and remarked that Dr. Adler would only make suggestions. The patient replied: 'Perhaps he will suggest something that will cure me,' and took his leave. Had this psychiatrist not been so obsessed with his desire to hinder the recognition of Individual Psychology he would certainly have noticed that he could not have kept the patient from coming to me and would have better understood the appropriateness of his remarks. I beg of you, my friends, when you are in the presence of patients avoid depreciatory remarks, even when they are justified. The open scientific arena is surely the place where wrong opinions should be corrected and replaced by views that are right; and this should be done by scientific methods.

If the patient at the first interview is in doubt as to whether he will undergo the treatment, leave the decision over until the next few days. The usual question about the duration of the treatment is not easy to answer. I consider this question quite justified, because a large number of those who visit me have heard of treatments that have lasted eight years and have been unsuccessful. Treatment by Individual Psychology, if properly carried out, must show at least a perceptible partial success in three months, in most cases even earlier. Since, however, success depends on the co-operation of the patient the correct procedure is to keep a door open for social feeling from the start by emphasizing the fact that the duration of the co-operation depends on the patient, that the physician, if he is well-grounded in Individual Psychology, can find his bearings after half an hour, but that he has to wait until the patient as well has recognized his style of life and its mistakes. Still one can add: 'If you are not convinced after one or two weeks that we are on the right path, I will stop the treatment.'

The unavoidable question of the fee causes difficulties. I have often received patients who have lost a not inconsiderable fortune in previous treatments. The consultant must bring himself into line with the fees customary in his district. He may also take into consideration any extra trouble and expenditure of time the case requires.

He should, however, abstain from making unusually large demands, especially when these would be harmful to the patient. Gratuitous treatment should be carried through in such a tactful manner that poor patients will not feel that the consultant shows in any way a lack of interest in their case. In most cases they never fail to notice this. The payment of a lump sum, even when that seems acceptable, or a promise to pay after a successful cure, should be declined, not because the latter is uncertain, but because it artificially introduces a new motive into the relationship between the doctor and his patient, and this makes successful treatment difficult. Payment should be made weekly or monthly, and always at the end of the period. Demands or expectations of any kind always do harm to the treatment. Even trivial kindly services which the patient quite often himself offers to give must be refused. Gifts should be declined in a friendly manner, or their acceptance postponed until after the cure has been completed. There should be no mutual invitations or joint visits during the treatment. The treatment of relatives or of persons known to the consultant is of a rather more difficult complexion, because in the nature of things any feeling of inferiority becomes more oppressive in the presence of an acquaintance. The person who has to deal with the case, too, is also averse to tracing his patient's feeling of inferiority, and he has to do his very utmost to make the patient feel at his ease. Any tension is greatly relieved when one has the good fortune, as in Individual Psychology, to be able in the treatment always to draw attention only to errors and never to innate defects, always to show that there is the possibility of a cure and make the patient feel that he is just as important as any one else, and always to point to the universally low level of social feeling. This helps us also to understand why Individual Psychology has never seen traces of the great 'resistance' that other systems have found. It is easy to see that the treatment in Individual Psychology never comes to a crisis, and when an Individual Psychologist not thoroughly well-grounded, say like Künkel, considers that crises—a shock or remorse on the part of the patient—are necessary, then the reason is simply that he has induced them to begin with, artificially and superfluously. It may be, too, because he is under the erroneous impression that he is thereby doing the Church a good turn.[1] I have always considered it a great advantage to keep the level of tension in the treatment as low as possible, and I have frankly developed a method of saying to almost every patient that there are jocular situations that are almost completely similar in structure to his particular neurosis, and therefore that he can take his trouble more lightly than he is doing. As for those critics who are rather dense, at the risk of being redundant I must take the word from their lips and add that, of course, such jocular allusions will not lead to the revival of the feeling of inferiority (which Freud at present finds so extraordinarily enlightening). References to fables and historical personages, and quotations from the poets and philosophers, help to

[1] cf. Jahn und Adler, *Religion und Individualpsychologie* (Verlag Dr. Passer, Vienna, 1933).

strengthen the belief in Individual Psychology and in its conceptions.

At every interview it ought to be noted whether or not the patient is on the way to co-operation. Every gesture, every expression, the material for discussion he brings with him or has not brought with him, will supply proof of this. A thorough understanding of dreams gives at the same time the opportunity of taking account of success or failure and of the amount of co-operation. But special caution must be exercised in spurring the patient on towards any particular line of action. If there should be any talk about this the doctor should not say anything for or against, but, ruling out as a matter of course all undertakings that are generally considered dangerous, he should tell the patient that, while he was convinced that he would be successful, he was not quite able to judge precisely whether he was really ready for the venture. Any incitement given before the patient has acquired a greater social feeling revenges itself as a rule by a strengthening or a recurrence of the symptoms.

Stronger measures may be taken when it comes to the question of a vocation. This does not in any way mean that the patient should be ordered to take up a profession, but simply that the consultant should point out to him that he is best prepared for a particular calling, and that he will most likely be successful in following it. As on the whole at every stage of the treatment, here also we must keep strictly to the method of encouraging the patient. We must act on the conviction of Individual Psychology—which has made so many unstable and vain people feel that their toes have been trodden on—viz. 'that' (apart from outstanding, special achievements about whose structure we can say very little) 'every one can do anything.'

With regard to the examination of a child who is on his first visit to the consultant, I consider the questionnaire which I and my collaborators have outlined, to be the best among all I have seen up till now. I append it here. Certainly only those will be able to handle it correctly who are possessed of adequate experience, who have an accurate knowledge of the views of Individual Psychology in their iron framework, and who have had sufficient practice in the art of guessing. In its use they will once again perceive that the whole art of understanding human characteristics consists in comprehending the individual's style of life that has been completed in childhood, in grasping the influences that were at work when the child was forming it, and in seeing how this style of life unfolds itself in grappling with the social problems of humanity. To the questionnaire, which was framed some years ago, it should be added that the degree of aggression—the activity—has to be noted; and it ought not to be forgotten that the vast majority of childish mistakes are due to the pampering that continuously intensifies the child's emotional struggle and thus leads him constantly into temptation. He is in this way so allured by enticements of the more varied kinds that he finds it difficult to resist, especially when he is in bad company.

QUESTIONNAIRE FOR INDIVIDUAL
PSYCHOLOGISTS

For the understanding and treatment of difficult children. Compiled and annotated by the International Society for Individual Psychology.

1. How long have the troubles lasted? In what situation was the child, materially and mentally, when the failings became noticeable?

(The following are important: changes in surroundings, starting school, change of school, change of teacher, birth of younger members of the family, setbacks at school, new friendships, illnesses of the child or of the parents, etc.)

2. Was there anything unusual about the child previously? Due to bodily or mental weakness? Cowardice? Carelessness? Desire to be alone? Clumsiness? Jealousy? Dependence on others at meals, in dressing, washing, going to bed? Is he afraid of being left alone? Afraid of darkness? Has he a clear idea of his sex? Any primary, secondary, and tertiary sexual characteristics? How does he regard the other sex? How far has his instruction in

sexual questions proceeded? Step-child? Illegitimate? Boarded out? What were his foster-parents like? Is he still in touch with them? Has he learned to walk and speak at the normal time? Does he do this without mistakes? Was the teething normal? Had he any noticeable difficulties in learning to write, calculate, draw, sing, swim? Has he had any special attachment to any one—mother, father, grandparents, nurse?

(Care should be taken to discover the establishment of a hostile attitude to life, anything that might rouse feelings of inferiority, tendencies to exclude difficulties and persons, traits of egotism, irritability, impatience, heightened emotion, activity, eagerness, caution.)

3. Has the child caused much trouble? What things or persons does he fear most? Does he cry out at night? Does he wet his bed? Does he want to domineer? Over strong, or only over weak persons? Has he shown a particular fondness for lying in the bed of one of his parents? Is he awkward? Intelligent? Was he much teased and laughed at? Does he show excessive vanity about his hair, clothing, shoes? Does he pick his nose? Bite his nails? Is he greedy at table? Has he stolen anything? Has he difficulties at the stool?

(This will show clearly whether he has given evidence of more or less activity in striving for pre-eminence. Further, whether obstinacy has prevented the cultivation of his instinctive activity.)

4. Did he make friends easily, or was he unsociable, and did he torment people and animals? Does he attach himself to younger persons, older, girls (boys)? Is he

inclined to take the lead? Or does he stand aside? Does he collect things? Is he niggardly? Fond of money?

(This will show his ability to make contact with other persons, and the extent to which he is discouraged.)

5. How does the child conduct himself at present in all these relationships? How does he behave at school? Does he attend willingly? Does he arrive too late? Is he agitated before going to school; does he hurry? Does he lose his books, satchel, and papers? Does he get excited about school tasks and examinations? Does he forget or refuse to do his home-lessons? Does he waste his time? Is he grubby? Indolent? Has he much or little concentration? Does he disturb the lessons? Attitude to his teacher? Critical? Arrogant? Indifferent? Does he seek help from others in his work, or does he always wait for them to make the offer? Is he keen about gymnastics and sport? Does he consider himself partly or entirely devoid of talent? Does he read a great deal? What sort of reading does he prefer? Is he backward in every subject?

(These questions will give an insight into the child's preparation for school life and into the results of experiments at school on the child. They will also show his attitude towards difficulties.)

6. Correct information regarding his home conditions, illnesses in the family, alcoholism, criminal tendencies, neurosis, debility, syphilis, epilepsy, standard of living? What deaths have there been? How old at the time? Is the child orphaned? Who rules in the family? Is the upbringing strict, fault-finding, pampering? Are the chil-

dren frightened at life? How are they looked after? Step-father or mother?

(This gives a view of the child in his position in the family and enables an estimate to be made of the influences that have helped to form the child.)

7. What is the place of the child in the family succession? Is he the oldest, second, youngest, or an only child? Any rivalries? Frequent crying? A spiteful laugh? Tendency to depreciate other persons without cause?

(Important for characterology; throws light on the child's attitude to other persons.)

8. What kind of ideas has the child at present about his future calling? What does he think about marriage? What are the professions of the other members of the family? What are the marital relations of his parents?

(From the answers it is possible to draw conclusions about the child's courage and his hope for the future.)

9. Favourite games? Favourite stories? Favourite characters in history and poetry? Is he fond of interrupting the games of other children? Does he become lost in fantasies? Day-dreams?

(This indicates his prototypes in his striving for superiority.)

10. Earliest recollections? Impressive or frequently recurring dreams? (Of flying, falling, being hindered, arriving too late for a train, running a race, being imprisoned, anxiety dreams.)

(One often finds in these a tendency to isolation; warning voices that lead the child to take excessive caution; ambitious impulses and the preference for certain persons, for passivity, etc.)

11. In what respect is the child discouraged? Does he feel himself slighted? Does he react favourably to appreciation and praise? Has he superstitious notions? Does he retreat from difficulties? Does he begin to do various things and then soon leave them alone? Is he uncertain about his future? Does he believe in the injurious effects of heredity? Was he systematically discouraged by those around him? Has he a pessimistic outlook on life?

(This will give important viewpoints for discovering whether the child has lost confidence in himself and is seeking his path in a wrong direction.)

12. Additional faults: Does he make grimaces? Does he behave himself stupidly, childishly, comically?

(Rather uncourageous attempts to draw attention to himself.)

13. Has he defects in speech? Is he ugly? Ungainly? Club-footed? Rickets? Knock-kneed or bow-legged? Badly developed? Abnormally stout, tall, small? Defects in the eyes or the ears? Is he mentally arrested? Left-handed? Does he snore at night? Is he strikingly good-looking?

(Here we are dealing with difficulties in life which the child as a rule exaggerates. These may lead to a chronic state of discouragement. A similar mistaken development often occurs in the case of very handsome children. They get the idea that everything must be given them to be retained without effort and in this way they neglect to make the right preparation for living.)

14. Does the child speak openly of his lack of ability, of his 'not being gifted enough' for school, for work, for life? Has he thoughts of suicide? Is there any connection in point of time between his want of success and his mistakes? (Neglect, forming gangs.) Does he place too great value on material success? Is he servile? Hypocritical? Rebellious?

(These are expressive forms of a deep-seated discouragement. They often occur after vain attempts to excel which have come to grief not only on account of their inherent aimlessness, but also as the result of want of understanding on the part of those round the child. After the failure there comes the search for a substitutive gratification in another field of struggle.)

15. The child's positive achievements? Type? Visual, acoustic, kinaesthetic?

(An important finger-post, since possibly the interest, inclination and preparation of the child point in another direction than that formerly taken.)

On the basis of these questions, which should not be put point by point, but conversationally, never mechanically, but always naturally and progressively, there is always formed a picture of the child's personality. By this the child's errors, though they are certainly not justified, will be made quite intelligible. When mistakes are discovered they should always be explained in a friendly manner, patiently and without threats.

In connection with the mistakes of adults I have found

the following model of examination to be of some value. By adhering to it the expert will gain well within half an hour a penetrating insight into the individual's style of life.

Certainly my own inquiries do not always keep to the rule of the following sequence. The expert will not fail to notice its agreement with a medical questionnaire. By following it the Individual Psychologist, on account of the system by which he works, will gain from the answers many a hint that would otherwise have remained unnoticed. The following is approximately the sequence:

1. What are you complaints?

2. How were you situated when you noticed your symptoms?

3. How are you situated now?

4. What is the nature of your calling?

5. Describe your parents in relation to their character, health, the illness of which they died, if they are not alive; what was their relation to yourself?

6. How many brothers and sisters have you? How are you placed among them? What is their attitude towards you? How are the others placed in life? Do they also have any illness?

7. Who was your father's or your mother's favourite?

8. Look for signs of pampering in childhood (timidity, shyness, difficulties in forming friendships, disorderliness, etc.).

9. Illnesses and attitude to illnesses in childhood?

10. Earliest recollections of childhood?

11. What do you fear, or what did you fear the most?

12. What are your ideas about the other sex, in childhood or in later years?

13. What calling would have most interested you, and in the event of your not having adopted it, why did you not do so?

14. Ambitious, sensitive, inclined to angry outbursts, pedantic, domineering, shy, impatient?

15. What sort of persons are around you at present? Impatient? Bad-tempered? Affectionate?

16. How do you sleep?

17. Dreams? (Of falling, flying, recurrent dreams, prophetic, about examinations, missing a train, etc.)

18. Illnesses in the family tree?

I should like at this point to give my readers an important hint. Any one who has come thus far and has not completely grasped the significance of these questions ought to begin again from the start and reflect whether he has not read this book with a lack of proper attention, or—God forbid!—with a hostile bias. If I had to explain here the meaning of these questions for our knowledge of the formation of the style of life, I should have to repeat the whole book. So this sequence of questions and the children's questionnaire may very well serve as a test, since the result will show whether the reader has gone along with me, that is, whether he has acquired an adequate amount of social feeling. That, indeed, is the most important object of this book. It is meant to

INDIVIDUAL PSYCHOLOGISTS

enable the reader not only to understand other persons, but to grasp the importance of social feeling and to make it living for himself.

INDEX

INDEX

INDEX

INDEX

CPSIA information can be obtained at www.ICGtesting.com
Printed in the USA
BVOW020038261111

276780BV00002B/106/P